SUPER FOODS
SUPER FAST

SUPERFOODS
SUPERFAST

100 ENERGIZING RECIPES TO MAKE IN 20 MINUTES OR LESS

JULIE MONTAGU
THE FLEXI FOODIE

Photography by Yuki Sugiura

Q

quadrille

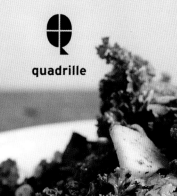

Contents

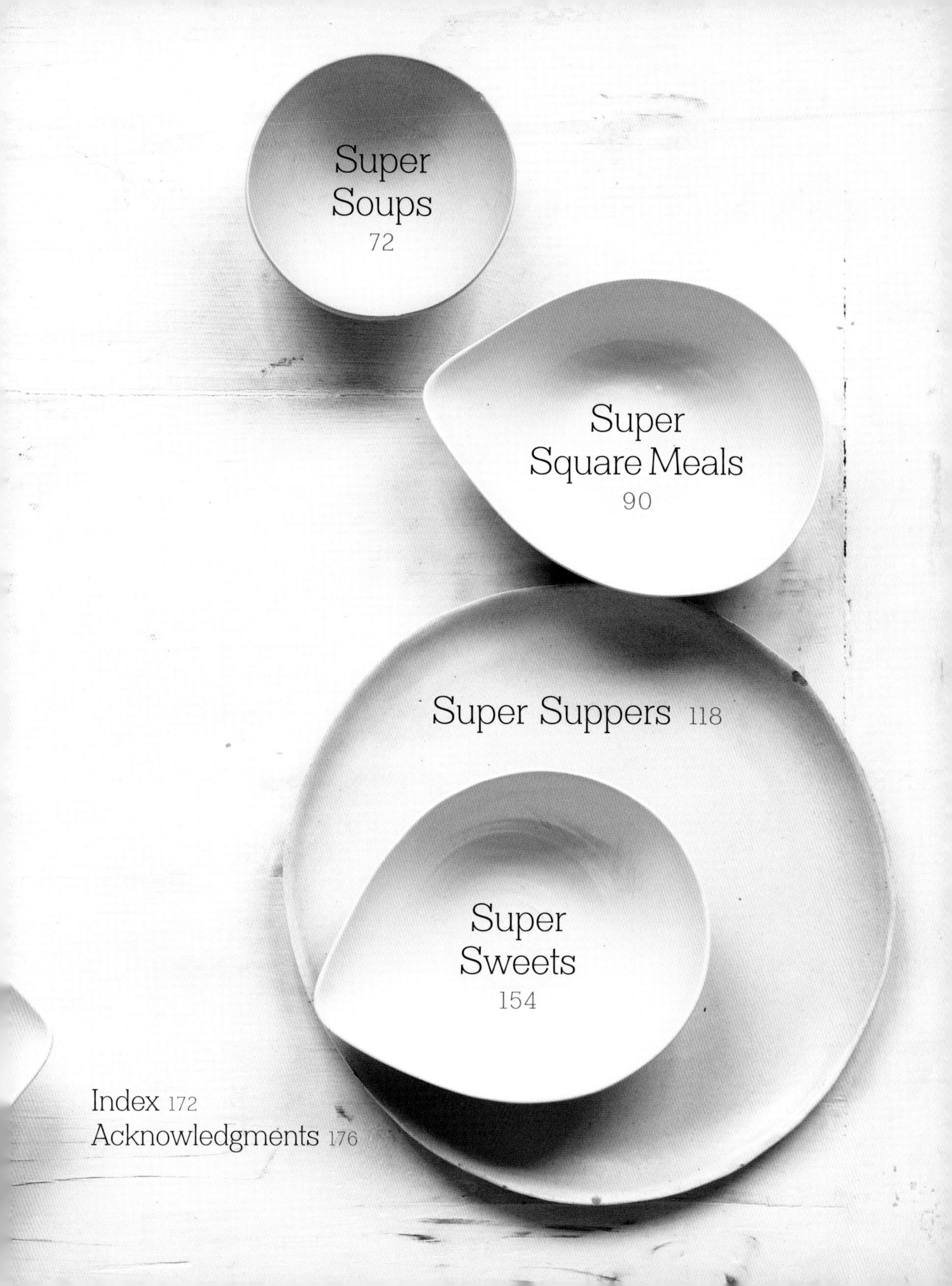

About this book

So, why this book? Why super – and why fast?! If you have my first cookbook *Superfoods*, you'll know that I introduced you to the superhero foods in each recipe. But some of those recipes take a bit of time to make and have quite a few ingredients – perfect for those days when you have a little breathing space and can slow down. Slowing down – now that's a good thing! But if you're anything like me and you have a hectic lifestyle (four kids and working full-time I think qualify as hectic!) but you still want to nourish your body and energize your mind so that you can keep going and going, then this book is for you busy people. Ask yourself this: do you ever feel hectic, crazy, overwhelmed, exhausted, overworked and well, just plain old busy? – then I mean you! Being busy is many people's excuse for not eating healthily and not taking care of themselves. That used to be me, too. This book is here to help YOU. So, in order to get the best out of it, here is my advice.

Most of the recipes in this book take well under 20 minutes to make, therefore they're super easy and the best bit is that they will make you feel great and energized. I like to think of these recipes and in particular the nutrients in the recipes as working hard to supply you with a surge of goodness and energy. I made sure of that! For this reason alone, it's worth giving yourself 20 minutes in the kitchen every day for the positive effect it will have on your wellbeing.

There are just a couple of recipes that require you to soak something (e.g. nuts) the night before but once that's done, the recipes take no time at all.

There are several recipes that will take exactly 20 minutes on the dot (I've timed them all!). In order to do this, please make sure that you have collected all the ingredients beforehand and that they are collected in front of you along with any utensils and measuring devices needed. As long as you are prepared and you don't have to go searching for anything while cooking, these recipes are 20 minutes from start to finish.

You will be multi-tasking in a number of recipes, of course, and I always try to make this clear. For example, while brown rice is cooking, you might need to be chopping veggies, sautéing onions and/or whisking a dressing. Speaking of which, brown rice *can* be cooked in under 20 minutes – the trick is to keep the water boiling at all times (something I learned from a dear friend). Oh, and when you're chopping veggies or any ingredient, roughly chopped is just fine.

That's it! That's all you busy people need to know in order to use this book effectively so that your body gets nourished and energized in 20 minutes or less.

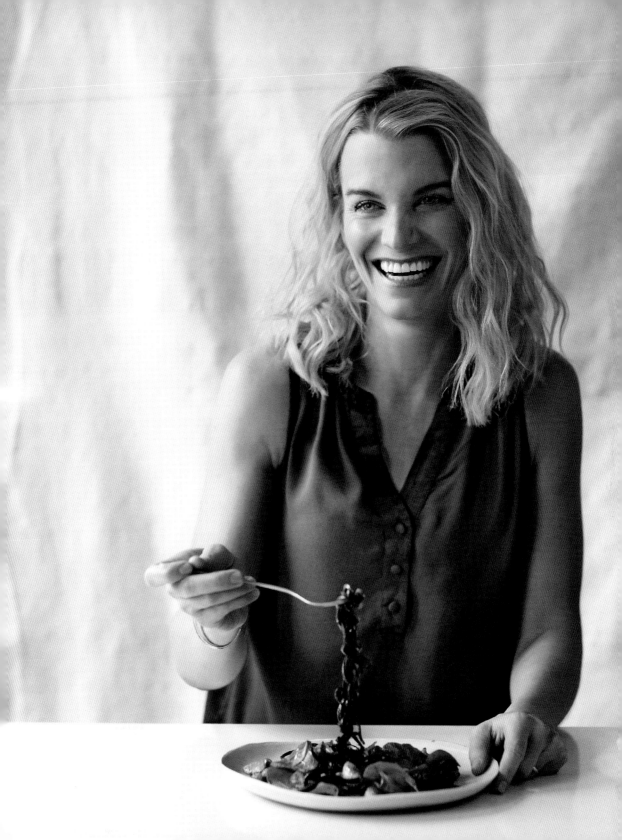

superYOU meal plans

Are you a commuter, an athlete, a working parent, a world traveller, a single guy or girl, a working couple, an exhausted parent, a student or an astronaut? Well, if you are one of these, then congratulations! Not only is this book for you, but I've laid out some meal plans, too, just to help you with your busy lives. Trust me, if you're anything like me, you'll need all the nutritional help you can get! So here are my top tips and meal plans for your busy lives.

When it comes to health, many busy people often wait until a problem arises before addressing it. However, through various lifestyle and dietary choices, we have the ability to work to prevent these issues in the first place. Adopting a lifestyle – even when we are super busy – that is effectively a preventative measure against disease gives us much more control over our health and our longevity. Instead of relying on modern medicines to intervene when we become ill, why shouldn't we take full responsibility for our body and mind through the actions, decisions and food we make every day?

By altering our diet, exercise regime, sleeping habits and stress levels for the better, we can encourage our body to bypass ill health.

These are my simple guidelines that everyone can easily adopt in order to live a life that promotes optimum health, both physical and mental, even when you are SUPER busy!

1. Embrace cooking as a necessary activity that enables your body to get all the nutrients that it needs. Choose real foods, and by that I mean fresh, organic when possible, wholesome foods that are not pumped full of chemicals and toxins. Find time every day to prepare your own meals even if they're quick, and be sure to get creative in order to keep yourself inspired. Food is one of the best preventative medicines we can administer ourselves and a healthy diet will aid a healthy body and mind.

2. Be sure to move each and every day. This doesn't mean you have to spend hours in the gym. You can choose to go for a walk in the morning, afternoon or evening – even just for 10 minutes – or cycle to work, to the store or to another mode of transport. Just make sure you are moving and stretching throughout your day. Not only will moving keep you physically healthy but it will also assist in combatting stress, reducing anxiety and improving your sleep.

3. Try to ensure that all your interactions with others are meaningful, respectful and positive. Work to strengthen your existing relationships and to form new connections with like-minded people who will bring happiness into your life. If you are aware that you have toxic relationships with certain people (I call them 'energy vampires'), then either talk it out and remedy the situation, or distance yourself from these people entirely. It is natural to seek the validation of others, however, it is not something that we really need in order to be happy. You will find that those who truly love you will bring you joy and not negativity. Evaluate your relationships and make it a priority to deepen your positive connections while eradicating the negative.

4. Be consciously grateful for the amazing aspects of your life and be sure to show it! Tell the people you care about that you care about them, have respect for your career, your home and your family, and affirm these facts in your mind. I find it helpful to list five things that I am grateful for each day as I wake and right before I fall asleep. These can be huge things, such as being alive, or relatively small things, such as being grateful for a delicious meal during the day. Showing thanks for the things you appreciate helps to reiterate how your life is on track, even when it doesn't feel like it.

5. I've picked my favourite fastest recipes for those weeks that you are insanely busy. Because at these times we often choose foods carelessly; they're last on the list of priorities and we tend to "grab & go" foods that our body is not happy about. So use these meal plans for the weeks when you have a lot on your plate but you know you just want and most certainly need to feel great.

Week ONE Meal Plan

MONDAY
Sunrise: Quinoa Seeded Breakfast in a Jar: page 22
Snack: Spacamole: 34
Square Meal: Burrito Salad Jar: page 102
Supper: Kale Mac and Cheese: page 124

TUESDAY
Sunrise: Avocado and Lime Yogurt Toast with Chilli: page 18
Snack: Cacao Snack Balls: page 38
Square Meal: Walnut and Black Bean Wraps: page 116
Supper: Spicy Butter Bean Dhal: page 120

WEDNESDAY
Sunrise: Coconut Oat Pudding: page 23
Snack: Spicy Macadamia Dip: page 36
Square Meal: Tabbouleh with Edamame and Pomegranate: page 108
Supper: Green Risotto: page 134

THURSDAY
Sunrise: Fruity Turmeric Breakfast Bowl: page 24
Snack: Cayenne and Lime Sunflower Seeds: page 30
Square Meal: Tostadas with Herb Hummus: page 96
Supper: Julie's Sloppy Joes: page 142

FRIDAY
Sunrise: Millet and Chia Porridge: page 26
Snack: Walnut Chia Bites: page 37
Square Meal: Curried Couscous: page 95
Supper: Perfect Pasta Primavera: page 144

Week TWO Meal Plan

MONDAY
Sunrise: Apple and Maple Buckwheat Stew in a Jar: page 22
Snack: Spicy Snack Balls: page 38
Square Meal: Spicy Noodle Jar: page 99
Supper: Spicy Tofu Tacos: page 140

TUESDAY
Sunrise: Tofu and Black Bean Corn Tortilla Wraps: page 27
Snack: Raw Chocolate Maca Truffles: page 37
Square Meal: Farro and Chickpea Stew: page 95
Supper: Cannellini Bean Masala: page 150

WEDNESDAY
Sunrise: Chocolate and Coconut Granola: page 16
Snack: Pumpkin Seed Pâté: page 32
Square Meal: Courgetti Spaghetti with Grapefruit and Brazil Nut Pesto: page 104
Supper: 3-Bean Spicy Chilli: page 122

THURSDAY
Sunrise: Vanilla Quinoa Porridge: page 26
Snack: Asparagus Fries (if have somewhere to heat this up, otherwise swap with another snack): page 40
Square Meal: Baked Chickpeas and Kale: page 112
Supper: Portobello Mushroom Burger with Red Pepper Sauce: page 126

FRIDAY
Sunrise: Superfood Chia Pudding: page 14
Snack: Nut Stuffed Mushrooms (if have somewhere to heat this up, otherwise swap with another snack): page 42
Square Meal: Fried Brown Rice with Tofu and Peanut Sauce: page 92
Supper: 'Cheesey' Polenta and Black-eyed Beans Stir Fry: page 128

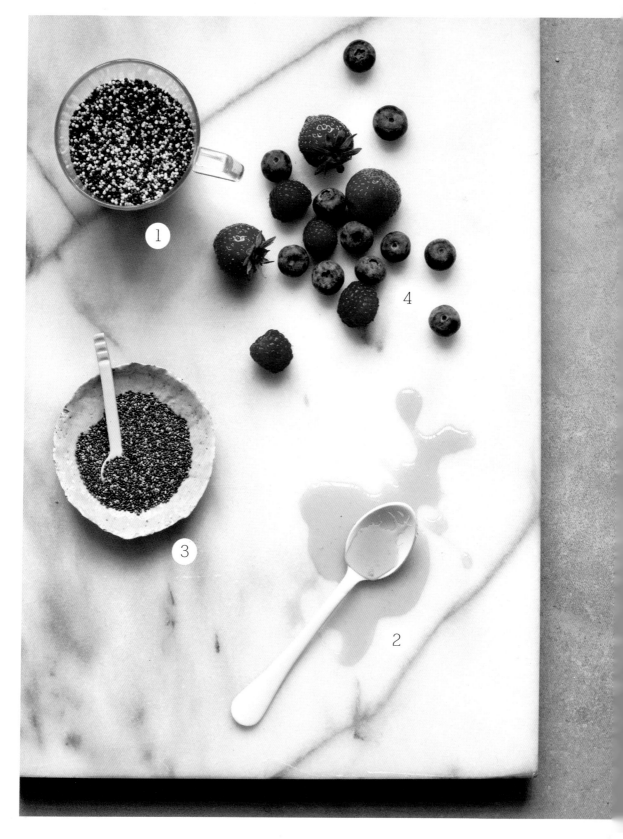

super SUNRISE

For a working mum of four, mornings are hectic to say the least!
I am always more worried about my kids getting their breakfasts
than I am about me! But I realized, after many years of NOT eating
breakfast, how grumpy and moody I became. Research has shown
that when we consume sugary breakfast cereals or pastries, our
blood sugar levels spike. Then excess insulin is produced and
within just a few short hours our blood sugar levels come crashing
back down, leaving us hungry again. Not only do we want to eat
again, but this is also likely to make us grumpy and agitated too.
For this reason it is best to eat a healthy wholefood breakfast,
and here are my favourite recipes for those crazy days. I've even
created three that you can take away with you if you're on the go.

superfood superheroes

1. Quinoa
Quinoa is a gluten-free seed that is packed
full of protein, fibre and minerals. Although
not technically a grain, it is often classed as a
whole grain and is one of the healthiest options
in this category. Its fibre content is twice that of
most other grains, which means great things for
your cholesterol, blood sugar levels and weight
management. Quinoa also contains all of the
essential amino acids, making it a fantastic
source of protein!

2. Honey
Honey is a natural combination of sugars,
water, minerals, vitamins, pollen and protein.
It also contains an abundance of important
vitamins such as vitamin B6, thiamine,
niacin and riboflavin, in addition to a host of
minerals such as potassium, zinc, magnesium,
iron, copper and calcium. Honey is also rich
in certain types of antioxidants, known as
flavonoids, which are amazing for reducing
free radical damage to cells!

3. Chia seeds
Chia seeds are without a doubt one of the
healthiest foods on the planet! They are packed
full of nutrients and are incredibly low in
calories. In fact, they are so tiny that they are
actually tasteless and can be added to virtually
any meal to increase its health benefits! Their
use throughout history can be traced back to
the Aztecs and the Mayans, the word 'chia'
meaning 'strength' in the Mayan language.

4. Berries – all berries
All berries are super healthy. They are high in
vitamin C and a great source of fibre. Not only
that, but they are also known to help boost the
immune system.

Superfood Chia Pudding

4 tablespoons chia seeds
125g (1 cup) blueberries,
  raspberries or strawberries,
  or a mixture
2 teaspoons raw cacao powder
2 teaspoons honey or maple
  syrup
1 teaspoon maca or lucuma
  powder
160ml (⅔ cup) nut milk

Serves 2

To be honest, chia seeds don't need to be soaked overnight, or even for a few hours. These tiny little powerhouse seeds absorb liquid right away and start to swell immediately. For me, 10 minutes is plenty of time to get these bad boys nice and gooey.

Mix all the ingredients together in a large bowl, reserving a few of the berries, and stir until well combined. You will notice that the chia seeds will soak up a lot of the nut milk. This should just take a few minutes and then just top with the remaining berries and it's ready to eat. Now that's quick!

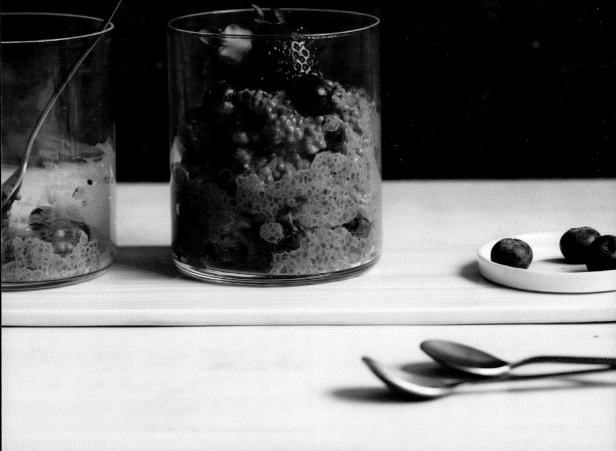

Chocolate and Coconut Granola

2 tablespoons coconut oil
65g (½ cup) blanched almonds
60g (½ cup) cashews
60g (½ cup) pecans
70g (½ cup) raisins
35g (¼ cup) sesame seeds
35g (¼ cup) pumpkin seeds
35g (¼ cup) unsweetened
   desiccated (dried) coconut
1 teaspoon raw cacao powder
1 teaspoon ground cinnamon
2 tablespoons honey
plant-based milk, to serve

Serves 4

Two of my four kids are obsessed with chocolate granola and, frankly, so am I! Let's be honest, it's actually hard to find a good, healthy version of chocolate granola, and when I have found it, it's VERY expensive. This recipe was invented with not only chocolate in mind, but also cost and time. So from my kitchen to yours, this one is simple, tastes so good and you can store it, too. Perfect.

Heat the coconut oil in a large frying pan over a medium heat. Add the nuts, raisins and seeds to the pan first, followed closely by the desiccated coconut, cacao powder, cinnamon and honey. Stir frequently for 15 minutes, reducing the heat slightly after 10 minutes.

Either serve yourself a portion with some plant-based milk and store the rest, or transfer everything to an airtight container.

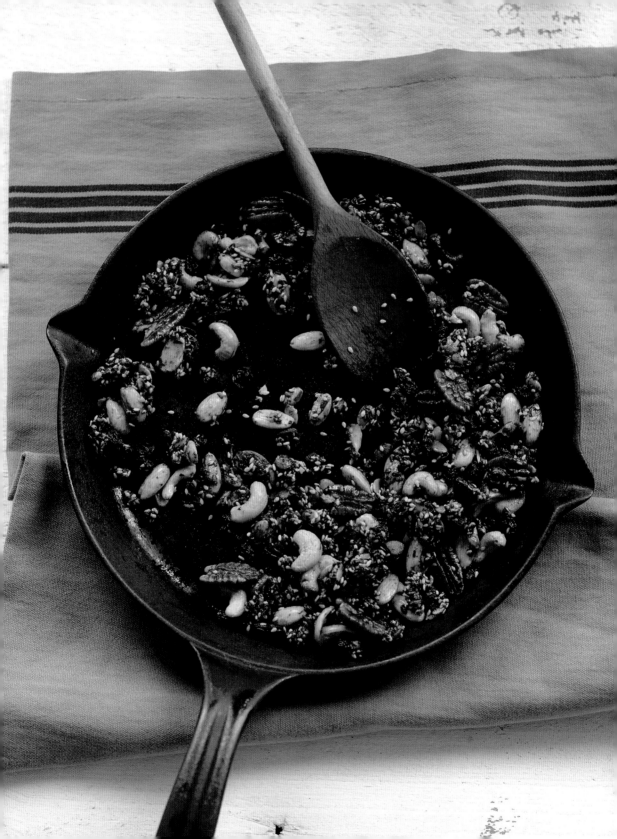

Avocado and Lime Yogurt Toast with Chilli

2 slices of bread (whatever
  kind you like – spelt, rye,
  gluten free)
1 avocado
good scoop of coconut or soya
  yogurt
zest and juice of 1 lime
1 teaspoon chilli flakes
  (red pepper flakes)
sea salt and freshly ground
  black pepper

Serves 2

Yes, another recipe for avocado on toast, but I mean, c'mon – it is SO good! I get that there are millions of pictures of avocado on toast all over your social media networks, but I still end up liking all of them because I love avocados so much. I think I could actually eat this breakfast every single day for the rest of my life, it's just too tempting. Plus it's a fun variation on your basic avo on toast.

Toast the bread while you slice open the avocado lengthways and remove the stone. Score the avocado length- and crossways, then scoop out the flesh with a spoon. Divide the avocado between the two pieces of toast and gently mash the flesh into the toast. Season with salt and pepper.

Place the yogurt in a bowl, squeeze in the lime juice and stir in the lime zest. Season with salt and pepper and mix to combine. Top each piece of avocado toast with the yogurt and sprinkle with the chilli flakes.

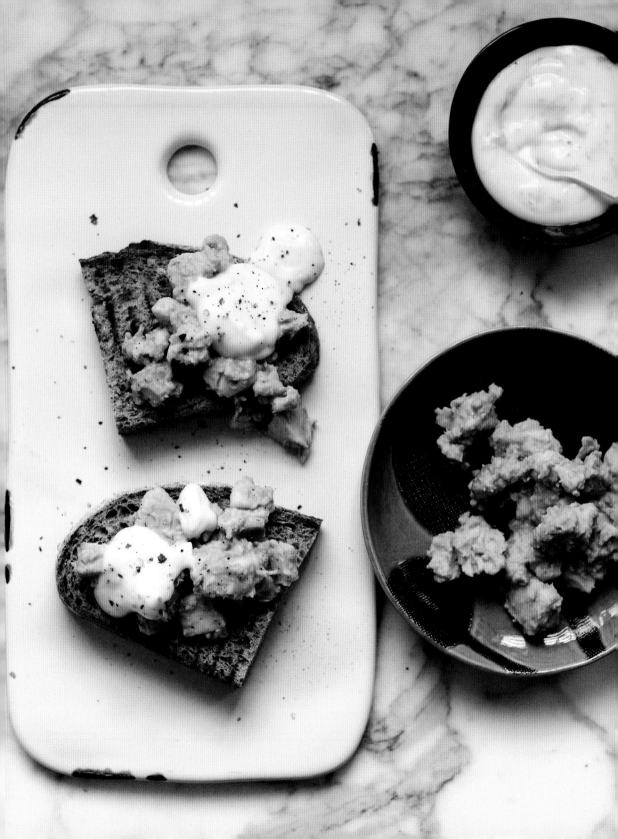

Breakfasts in a Jar

Raw Oatmeal with Chia Jam in a Jar

45g (½ cup) rolled oats
180ml (¾ cup) almond milk
  (or other nut or coconut milk)
½ teaspoon ground cinnamon
4 brazil nuts, chopped into
  small pieces (or other nuts)

For the Chia Jam
4 strawberries, chopped
1 tablespoon honey
1 teaspoon chia seeds
1 teaspoon lemon juice

1 jam jar, cleaned and dried

Serves 1

The following three recipes are designed to be made the night before when you know you have to get up early to catch a flight or get a child to an early morning school trip. You then have the jar in the fridge when you wake up – you just need to 'grab and go'. Of course, they take 20 minutes or less to make.

In a small saucepan over a medium-high heat, stir together the strawberries and honey for the jam. Once the strawberries start releasing their liquids (after about 10 minutes), mash them with a fork. Add the chia seeds and lemon juice and reduce the heat to low, allowing the seeds to swell and the jam to thicken (about 5 minutes). Remove from the heat.

Pour all the remaining ingredients and the chia jam into a jar and place in the fridge overnight. The raw oats will absorb the milk and all the delicious flavours.

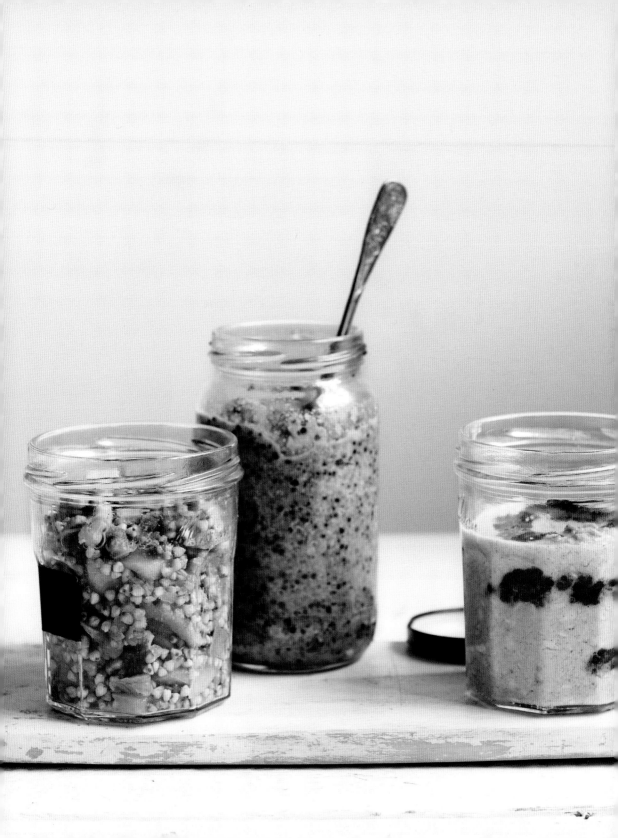

Quinoa Seeded Breakfast in a Jar

Apple and Maple Buckwheat Stew in a Jar

½ grapefruit, peeled, segmented and roughly chopped
1 fresh fig, chopped
120ml (½ cup) coconut milk
very small handful of pecans
45g (¼ cup) cooked quinoa (just follow the instructions on the packaging – it takes 15 minutes to cook)
1 teaspoon chia seeds
1 teaspoon ground flaxseed (linseed)
1 tablespoon honey

1 jam jar, cleaned and dried

Serves 1

Blend the grapefruit, fig, coconut milk and pecans in a blender, then add the cooked quinoa, seeds and honey and pour the mixture into a jar. Seal and leave overnight in the fridge.

It will be ready to go in the morning.

240ml (1 cup) coconut milk
55g (⅓ cup) buckwheat groats
1 apple, cored and chopped (keep the skin on!)
ground cinnamon, to taste
small handful of chopped walnuts
1 tablespoon maple syrup
sea salt

1 jam jar, cleaned and dried

Serves 1

Bring the coconut milk, buckwheat groats, apple pieces and a pinch of salt to the boil in a medium saucepan and let simmer for 15 minutes. Before the buckwheat has completely finished absorbing the milk, pour the mixture into a jar or Thermos and add the cinnamon, walnuts and maple syrup.

Put the lid on and leave out overnight to finish 'cooking'.

Coconut Oat Pudding

35g (⅓ cup) rolled oats
80ml (⅓ cup) coconut milk
60ml (¼ cup) water
1 teaspoon ground cinnamon
1 teaspoon maca or lucuma
  powder
1 fresh date, pitted and finely
  chopped
1 tablespoon unsweetened
  desiccated (dried) coconut
1 tablespoon raisins
1 tablespoon almonds,
  chopped

Serves 1

This breakfast pudding has just the right amount of sweetness – not so much to rapidly spike that blood sugar, but just enough to satisfy a sweet tooth AND keep blood sugar at a perfect level until lunchtime. Oh, and yes it's great that oats are a nutritional powerhouse, but I love them even more because they cook FAST! Just what I need for super-hectic mornings.

Place the oats, coconut milk, water, cinnamon, maca or lucuma powder and the chopped date into a small saucepan and cook over a medium heat until thick and creamy – this should take about 7 minutes.

Pour into a bowl and top with the shredded coconut, raisins and almonds.

Fruity Turmeric Breakfast Bowl

1 x 400ml tin (1¾ cups) coconut milk, refrigerated overnight
½ banana, roughly chopped
½ green apple, cored and roughly chopped
½ teaspoon ground ginger or grated fresh ginger
1 teaspoon ground or freshly grated turmeric
100g (1 cup) strawberries, chopped
100g (¾ cup) blueberries
honey, for drizzling

Serves 2

I think turmeric is one of the greatest spices we can add to our diets, especially because of its recently discovered link with fighting dementia. Ground turmeric is perfectly good, but grated fresh turmeric is even better. It's probably not possible to have a curry every night of the week, so I try to think of other ways to incorporate it into my diet. This one works a charm.

Spoon the cream off the top of the coconut milk and add the milk below to a food processor or blender with the banana, apple, ginger and turmeric. Blitz until smooth, then pour into bowls and top with the strawberries, blueberries and a drizzle of honey. That's all it takes – a super-easy way to get that super spice in!

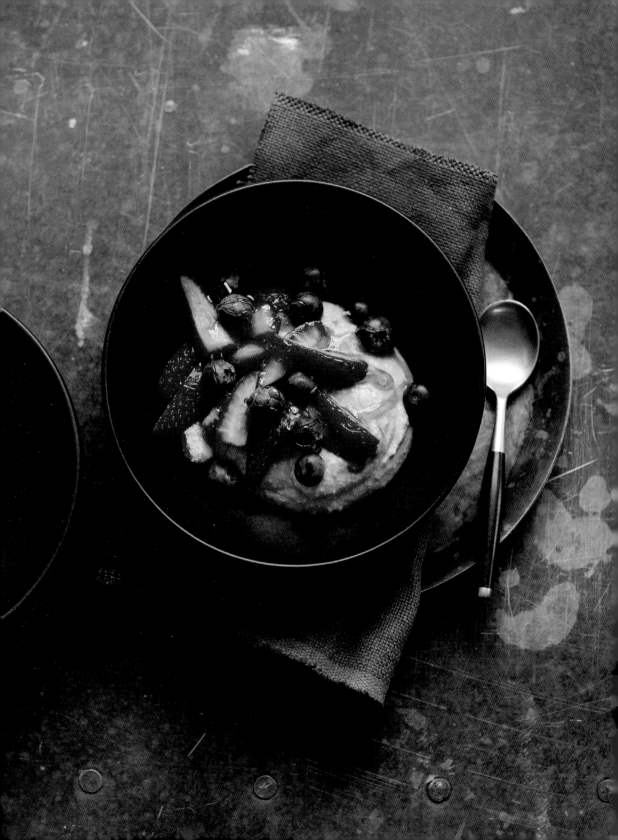

Millet and Chia Porridge

Vanilla Quinoa Porridge

Whole grains are great to get into your body early in the morning because they are packed with energy to keep you fuelled until your next meal. I like millet because, just like oats, it's going to keep my energy levels up without a mid-morning crash AND millet is super easy and fast to cook. Add in the chia and here's to a winning breakfast all round.

I've been addicted to vanilla since I was a kid. If I could put vanilla in everything, I seriously would! I particularly like this porridge on cold, dreary days because the vanilla combined with the cinnamon and nutmeg really warms me up. And when I'm warm on the inside, I'm definitely in a better mood when I take that first step out into the cold.

100g (½ cup) uncooked millet
100ml (⅓ cup + 1 tablespoon) coconut milk
40g (⅓ cup) cashews
1 teaspoon ground cinnamon
2 teaspoons chia seeds
2 tablespoons honey
mixed fresh fruit, optional

60g (⅓ cup) uncooked quinoa
240ml (1 cup) almond milk
1 teaspoon ground cinnamon
¼ teaspoon ground nutmeg
½ teaspoon vanilla extract
3 fresh dates, pitted and finely chopped
½ banana, sliced
maple syrup, for drizzling

Serves 2

Serves 1

Bring 400ml (1¾ cups) water to the boil in a medium saucepan and add the millet. Lower the heat and stir. As the water reduces, pour in the coconut milk and continue to stir. After a few more minutes, add the cashews and cinnamon. Leave to simmer on a low heat for 3–5 minutes and then spoon into bowls.

Combine the quinoa, almond milk, cinnamon, nutmeg, vanilla and chopped dates in a small saucepan over a medium heat and cook until creamy – this should take about 15 minutes.

Serve topped with the sliced banana and drizzled with maple syrup.

Top each bowl with a teaspoon of chia seeds, a tablespoon of honey and any fresh fruit you fancy.

Tofu and Black Bean Corn Tortilla Wraps

3 tablespoons olive oil
½ small red onion, chopped
½ red (bell) pepper, seeds
 removed and chopped
1 garlic clove, minced
225g (8 oz) extra-firm tofu,
 drained and crumbled
1 teaspoon ground coriander
1 teaspoon ground cumin
¼ teaspoon chilli (chili) powder,
 optional
200g (1¼ cups) black beans,
 drained and rinsed
handful of coriander (cilantro),
 roughly chopped
zest and juice of 1 lime
2 corn tortillas
large scoop of coconut or soya
 yogurt
sea salt and freshly ground
 black pepper

Serves 2

Think of this one as a much healthier alternative to Huevos Rancheros, yet in my opinion JUST AS GOOD! And if you're looking for protein in the morning, then look no further, as the tofu and black beans provide a hefty dose. This is one of my favourite breakfast recipes on a lazy weekend – well, before I chauffeur my kids around to their various activities!

Place a large frying pan over a medium-high heat and coat with the olive oil. Sauté the chopped onion and pepper for 2 minutes, or until soft. Add the garlic and cook for another minute. Add the crumbled tofu, ground coriander, cumin, chilli powder and a pinch of salt and pepper, and mix to combine. Sauté for a few minutes and then add the black beans. Mix together well and cook for another minute or so.

Remove the pan from the heat and add the fresh coriander and the lime zest and juice. Serve in the corn tortillas and top with a spoonful of yogurt.

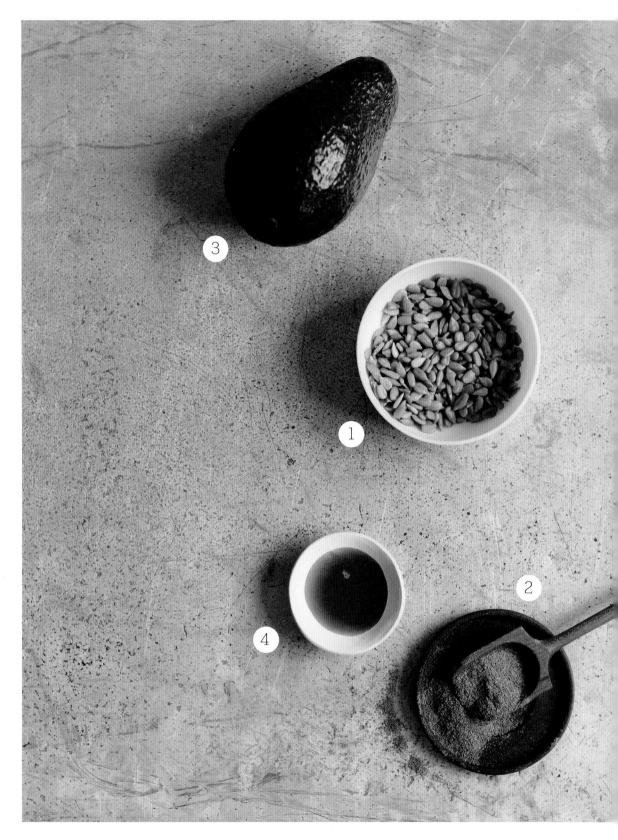

super SNACKS

Being on the go, non-stop running around, whether it's dropping off kids, collecting them and then taking them to their after-school activities, or commuting every day, rushing to meetings, making that plane or train, or simply being exhausted from working and doing too much! Believe me, I've been there many, many times and I know there will be many more in the future. But what I've learned is that it's great to have some yummy, delicious and 'good for you' snacks to energize you while you're rushing around. These snacks take very little time to make, so put your favourite song on for 4–5 minutes and dance around the kitchen while you make these Super Snacks and you'll not only be done in a flash, but your body will love you more for it!

superfood superheroes

1. Sunflower seeds
Sunflower seeds may be small but they pack a powerful nutritional punch! They contain exciting amounts of heart-healthy monounsaturated and polyunsaturated fats that make them useful for preserving cardiovascular health. Sunflower seeds are also rich in many essential vitamins and minerals that help to prevent disease and lower blood pressure.

2. Cumin
Cumin is known to aid digestion and boost immunity, and has also been linked to maintaining the health of the respiratory system. Early studies have also suggested that cumin could be useful in preventing the onset of diabetes by lowering the chances of hypoglycaemia.

3. Avocado
Avocados are incredibly rich in omega-3 fatty acids, which are beneficial for heart health. They are also high in protein while being low in natural sugars. They contain a wide range of vitamins and minerals and are especially useful for regulating the digestive system.

4. Maple syrup
Maple syrup is an incredible alternative to popular sweeteners because it is delicious and nutritious, too! It is a particularly excellent source of manganese, which is essential for keeping energy levels up. Manganese also helps the brain and nerves to function as they should. Additionally, maple syrup contains useful amounts of riboflavin, magnesium, zinc, calcium and potassium!

Cayenne and Lime Sunflower Seeds

Crunchy Cumin Chickpeas

Iron is such an important nutrient, but sadly so many of us simply do not consume enough of it. Sunflower seeds are a fantastic source and are an amazing snack food. As an added plus, lime is known to increase iron absorption in the body.

Possibly one of my favourite on-the-go snacks. Seriously. I am much more of a savoury person than a sweet one and so having a bag of these in my backpack while cycling around London is perfect, delicious and super energizing, which is exactly what I need.

150g (1¼ cups) sunflower seeds
1 teaspoon olive oil
juice of 1 lime
½ teaspoon cayenne pepper
½ teaspoon sea salt

Makes 3 servings

1 x 400g tin (1½ cups) chickpeas
  (garbanzo beans), drained and rinsed
1 tablespoon olive oil
½ teaspoon sea salt
1 teaspoon ground cumin
pinch of cayenne pepper, optional

Makes 6 good handfuls

Preheat the oven to 180°C/350°F/gas 4 and line a baking sheet with parchment paper.

Put the sunflower seeds into a bowl and coat with the olive oil, lime juice, cayenne pepper and salt. Spread the seeds on the baking sheet and bake for 15 minutes. Either serve immediately or leave to cool before storing in an airtight container.

Preheat the oven to 200°C/400°F/gas 6 and line a baking sheet with parchment paper.

Put the chickpeas into a bowl and coat with the olive oil, salt and spices before spreading them out on the baking sheet and roasting them for 15 minutes. Either serve immediately or leave to cool before storing in an airtight container.

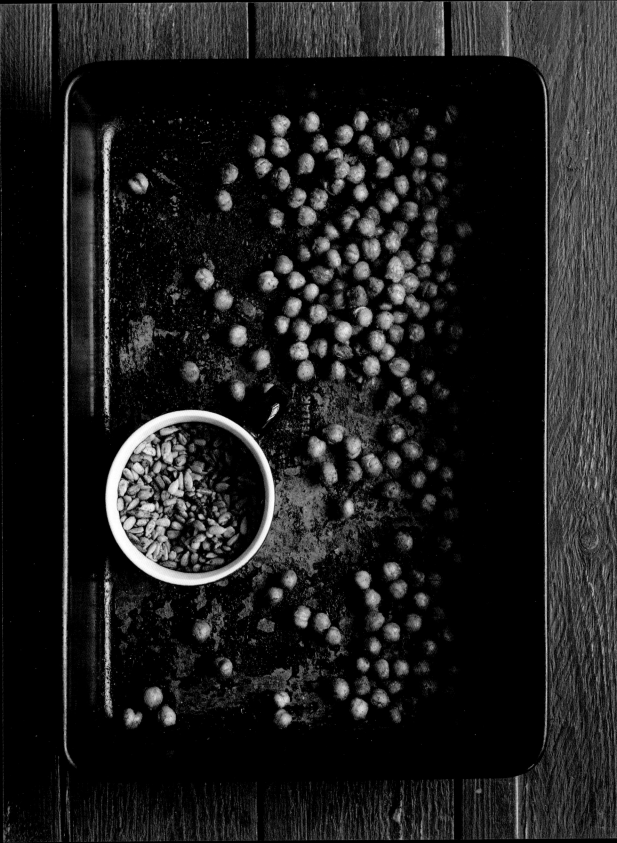

Pumpkin Seed Pâté

1 large celery stick, roughly chopped
1 spring onion (scallion), roughly chopped
1 large garlic clove
130g (1 cup) pumpkin seeds, soaked for 8 hours
2 tablespoons extra virgin olive oil
1 teaspoon dried oregano
¼ teaspoon sea salt
¼ teaspoon ground black pepper
zest and juice of 1 large lemon

Serves 3–4

I promise you, this is an amazing snack! And it's so, so easy to make. Put it in an airtight container and use it to top some large lettuce leaves (romaine and chicory work very well). Or spread on crackers and top with some yummy veggies such as sliced avocado or cucumber, radishes, shredded carrots or even sprouts.

Blend all the ingredients in a food processor or blender until well combined. Transfer to a bowl and serve, or store in an airtight container for a couple of days.

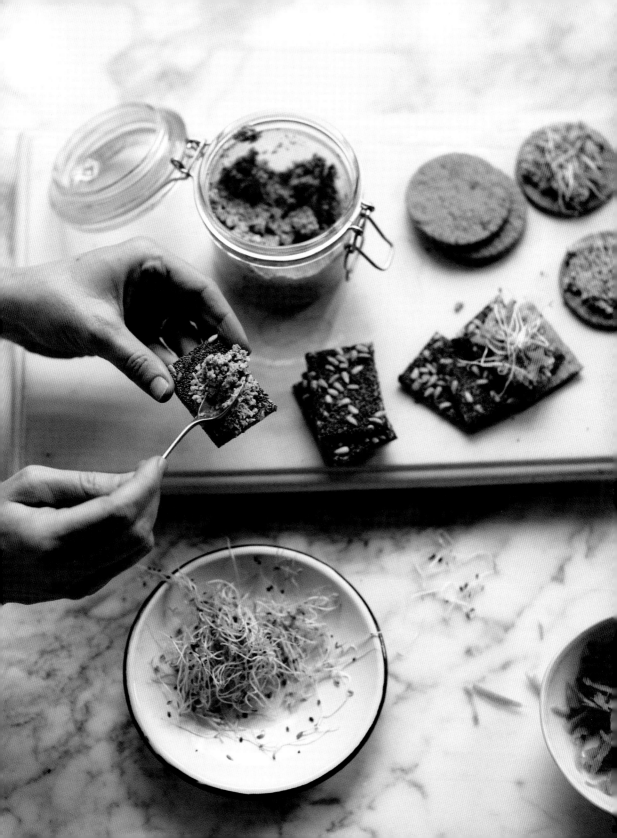

Spacamole

100g (¾ cup) frozen peas
1 avocado, peeled and stoned
handful of fresh spinach
juice of 1 lime
½ red chilli (chile pepper),
  chopped
small handful of coriander
  (cilantro)
¼ cucumber, roughly chopped
½ red onion, roughly chopped
vegetable sticks, for dipping

Serves 2

There's guacamole and then there's my Spacamole!
I try to add greens to as many dishes as I can – sort
of like trying to 'hide' them so people don't freak out.
And this is a perfect example. The lime will help stop
the avocado browning throughout the day, making it
super easy to take to work in a container along with
some carrots, cucumbers and radishes for dipping.

Fill a small pan with water and bring to the boil. Add
the peas and boil for 5 minutes. Drain and rinse well.

In a food processor or blender, blend the peas,
avocado, spinach, lime juice, chilli, coriander,
cucumber and red onion until smooth.

Put in a takeaway container with some vegetable sticks
for dipping and have yourself a perfect healthy snack.

Photographed with Spicy Macadamia Dip (see page 36).

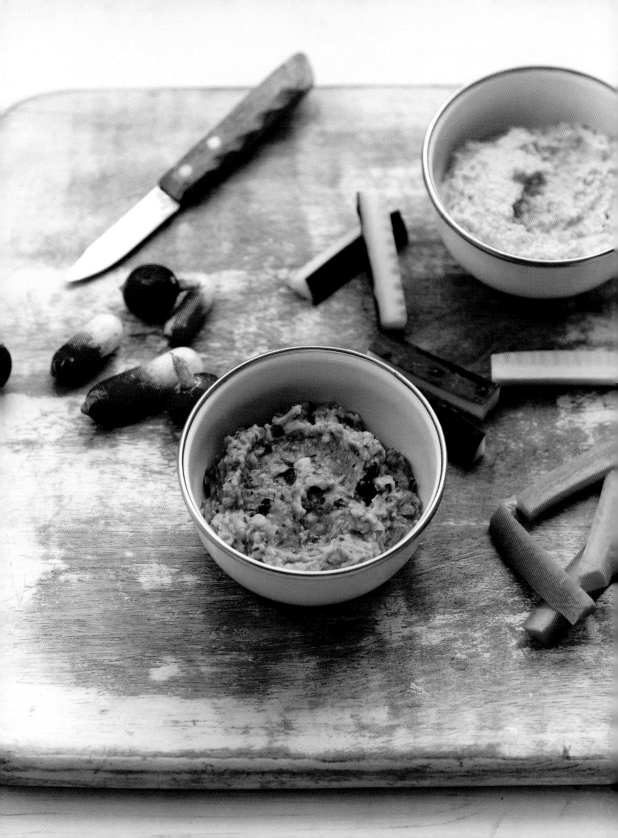

Spicy Macadamia Dip

100g (¾ cup) macadamia nuts
½ avocado, peeled and stoned
100ml (⅓ cup + 1 tablespoon)
   coconut milk
handful of basil
1 teaspoon chilli flakes
   (red pepper flakes)
juice of ½ lemon
sea salt and freshly ground
   black pepper
vegetables, for dipping

Serves 2

Grab some carrots, cucumber, radishes and cherry tomatoes and pack them in a bag along with this dip. Then you will be able to dip in and out of this amazingly creamy and yummy and, yes, good-for-you dip throughout your day. Whether at the office or travelling, this snack is the one that keeps going and going and going. If you don't have macadamia nuts, simply use cashews or walnuts, as they are also a good option for this delicious dip.

Blend all the ingredients in a food processor or blender until nice and smooth.

Place in an airtight container, along with a separate baggie filled with your choice of veggies, and you are good to go for healthy snacking all day long.

Photographed on page 35.

Walnut Chia Bites

Raw Chocolate Maca Truffles

Walnuts are my favourite nuts not only for their taste and the fact that I can use them in pretty much everything from salads to soups and smoothies – and these super snacks – but also because of the added bonus of Omega-3s that other nuts don't have. That's what makes walnuts super special.

50g (heaping ⅓ cup) walnut halves
12 fresh dates, pitted
70g (½ cup) unsweetened desiccated
  (dried) coconut
1 tablespoon chia seeds
1 tablespoon maple syrup

Makes 10

Preheat the oven to 220°C/425°F/gas 7 and roast the walnuts on a baking sheet for 10 minutes. Remove from the oven and blitz to a smooth paste in a food processor or blender with the rest of the ingredients.

Transfer to a bowl and use your hands to roll the mixture into 10 balls. Eat immediately or refrigerate for a few hours for a harder texture.

Maca is great for balancing stress hormones, decreasing stress levels and providing amazing energy and endurance. So these bad boys are perfect for those stressful days when you need just that extra little bit of oomph to make it through.

200ml (¾ cup + 1½ tablespoons) coconut milk
60g (½ cup) oats
50g (½ cup) maca powder
50g (½ cup) raw cacao powder
2 tablespoons maple syrup
1 teaspoon ground cinnamon

Makes 10–12

Blitz everything together in a food processor or blender. Transfer to a bowl and use your hands to roll the mixture into 10–12 balls. Refrigerate for 10 minutes to set.

Cacao Snack Balls

Calling all chocolate and nut lovers, these balls are for you! When I need to get my chocolate fix, this is my go-to recipe. Mix these guys up and just keep in your fridge for when you need a pick-me-up – grab one and watch your energy soar.

80g (heaping ⅔ cup) cashews
80g (scant ⅔ cup) walnut halves
4 tablespoons raw cacao powder,
   plus extra for dusting
4 tablespoons coconut oil
2 tablespoons honey
2 teaspoons chia seeds
2 teaspoons flaxseed (linseed)

Makes 10–12

Blitz everything together in a food processor or blender. Transfer to a bowl and use your hands to roll the mixture into 10–12 balls. Dust with cacao powder and refrigerate, ready to grab when you need a boost!

Spicy Snack Balls

I like spice. When I was younger, I always used to say, 'The spicier the better!' I'm also a big energy snack fan and I wanted to somehow incorporate my favourite spices into my favourite energy balls. That is exactly how these guys were created.

80g (⅔ cup) brazil nuts
20g (2½ tablespoons) sunflower seeds
10 fresh dates, pitted
4 tablespoons coconut oil
2 tablespoons honey
2 teaspoons chilli flakes (red pepper flakes)
2 teaspoons paprika
1 teaspoon ground ginger

Makes 10–12

Blitz everything together in a food processor or blender and then use your hands to roll into balls before refrigerating.

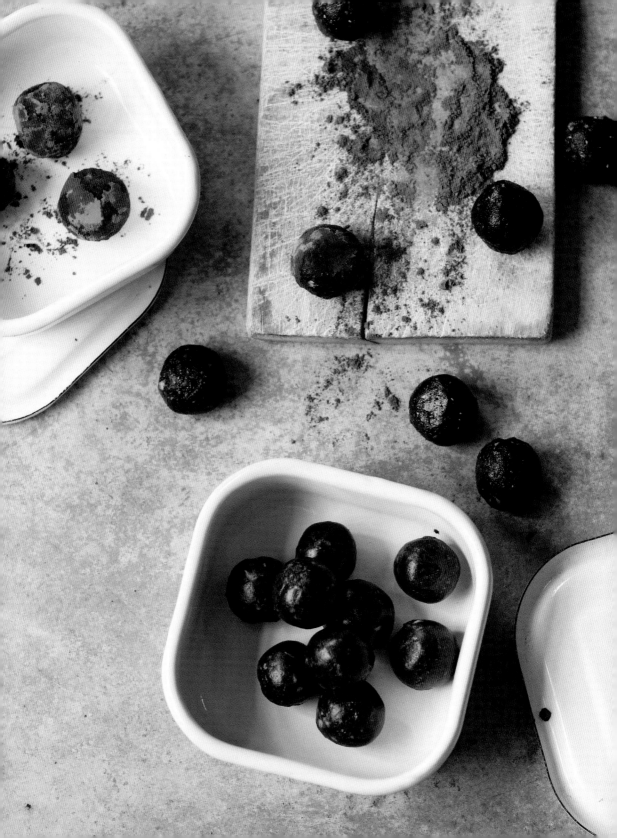

Asparagus Fries

100g (3½oz) asparagus spears,
  woody ends trimmed
2 tablespoons coconut oil,
  melted
1 teaspoon ground cumin
1 teaspoon paprika
2 tablespoons nutritional yeast
35g (½ cup) gluten-free
  breadcrumbs
sea salt and freshly ground
  black pepper

Makes 1–2 servings

We all know about courgette (zucchini) fries, French fries and sweet potato fries, but have you heard of asparagus fries? Well, I urge you to go and make these ASAP! And because asparagus is very often served cold, it makes these guys the ideal takeaway snack. Pretty perfect if you ask me!

Preheat the oven to 220°C/425°F/gas 7 and line a baking sheet with parchment paper.

In a bowl, coat the asparagus spears with the melted coconut oil, followed by the cumin, paprika, nutritional yeast, a good sprinkling of salt and pepper and the breadcrumbs. Spread them out on the baking sheet and sprinkle any of the mixture left in the bowl over the top. Bake for 15 minutes.

Serve immediately or allow to cool and eat them later in the day when you need an energizing snack.

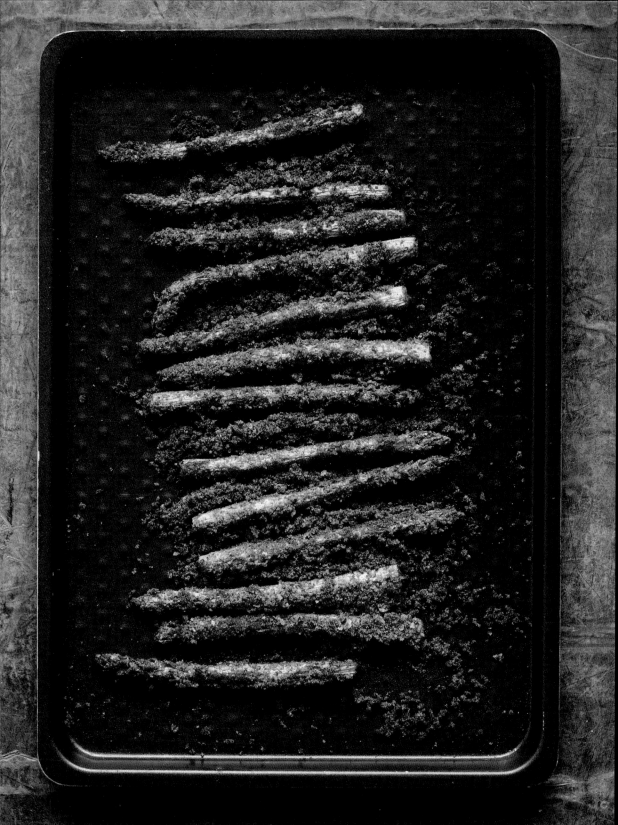

Nut-stuffed Mushrooms

30g (¼ cup) walnut halves,
  ground
30g (¼ cup) blanched almonds,
  ground
30g (scant ¼ cup) pumpkin
  seeds, ground
1 teaspoon smoked paprika
1 teaspoon dried oregano
4 tablespoons olive oil
4 large portobello mushrooms,
  stems and gills removed

Serves 4

When I'm working from home, this is my go-to snack every single time. I particularly like this when I need some brain food during my working day. Mushrooms are being hailed as the new kale because of their enormous health benefits and I believe it! So here's my brain food snack for those days when you really need a nutritional punch in the face…

Preheat the oven to 220°C/425°F/gas 7 and line a baking sheet with parchment paper.

Mix the ground nuts and seeds together in a bowl, add the paprika, oregano and olive oil and mix well. Place the mushrooms, cap side down, on the baking sheet and spoon equal amounts of the filling mixture onto each mushroom. Bake for 10–12 minutes before serving hot.

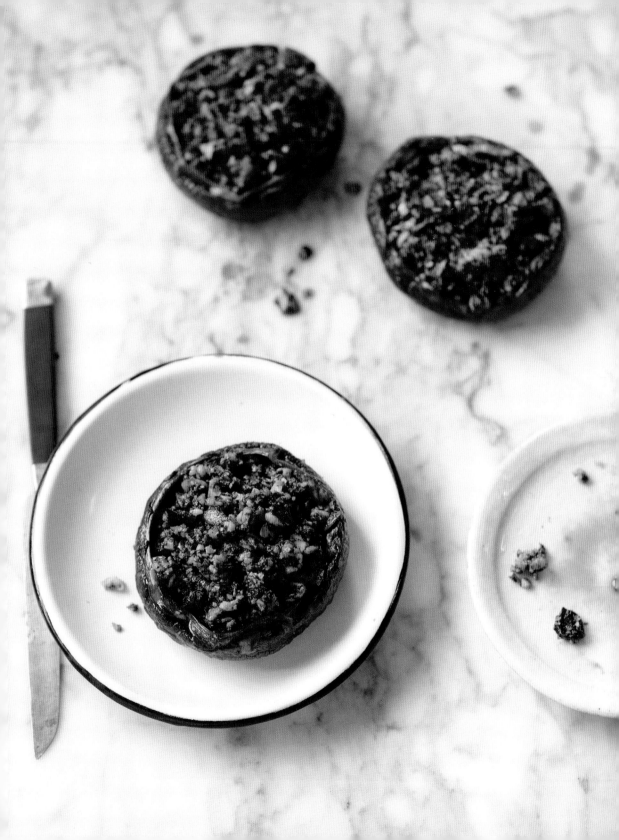

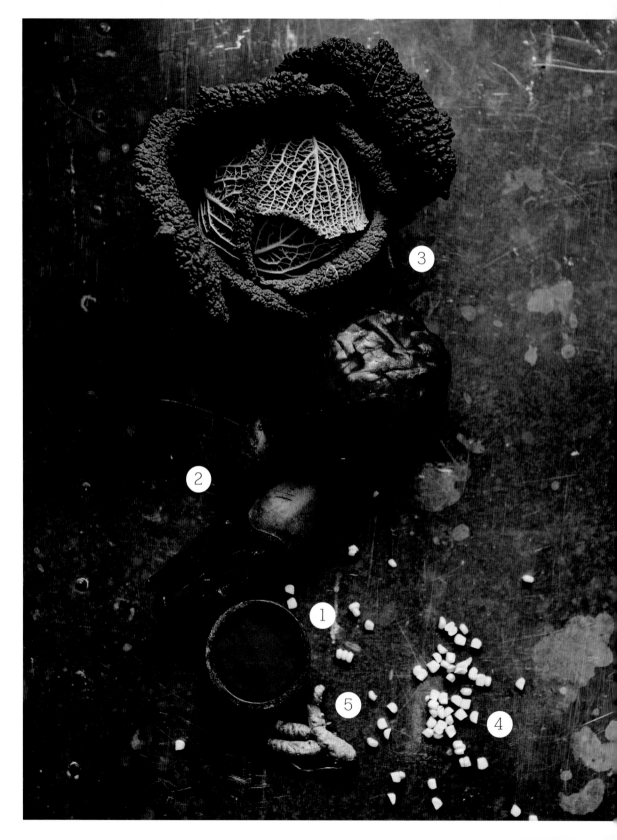

super SALADS

I have to say, my favourite thing in the world to make is salad. Why, you ask? Well, I love the fact that what we used to think of as a salad has evolved so much. Of course I love dark leafy greens and get them in my diet as much as I can, but that doesn't mean that every salad has to have some form of lettuce in it any more. Using legumes, beans, broccoli and even cauliflower as a base for a salad is, to me, just a bit more fun and a lot more creative. So here are some simple yet super-interesting and very tasty salads that you can easily pack up and take with you wherever you go. Add a couple of pieces of your preferred bread, too, for those days when you need a heartier meal!

superfood superheroes

1. Paprika
Paprika is the perfect spice for boosting the flavour (and colour) of a dish because of its spicy yet subtle taste. It should be embraced especially for its high antioxidant count. Paprika contains many vitamins and minerals, most notably vitamins A, B6 and iron.

2. Beetroot (Beets)
As well as being rich in vitamins and minerals, beetroot are also useful for cleansing the body. When eaten they work to purify the blood, which can help to protect the body against certain cancers. They are also believed to be beneficial for mental health because of the natural presence of betaine, a substance used in the treatment of depression.

3. Cabbage
Cabbage is great for lowering your cholesterol as well as helping to protect you against certain cancers. It is an impressive source of vitamin C and manganese, and contains high levels of a group of antioxidants known as polyphenols. Regular consumption of polyphenols is linked to a lower incidence of degenerative diseases.

4. Sweetcorn (Corn)
One of the great things about sweetcorn is that its antioxidant activity is actually heightened through cooking, unlike many other vegetables where the opposite is the case. In addition to this, it is full of lutein and zeaxanthin, both of which help to maintain healthy vision.

5. Turmeric
Turmeric has been prized throughout history for its medicinal uses and is particularly common in Indian cuisine. When consumed with black pepper, turmeric is much more easily absorbed into the bloodstream, helping the body to enjoy its health benefits. Not only is turmeric full of vitamins and minerals, but it is also naturally anti-inflammatory and works to promote optimum heart health.

Fennel and Pear Salad with Spicy Almonds and Avocado

large handful of blanched
   almonds
2 teaspoons coconut oil, melted
1 teaspoon cayenne pepper
1 fennel bulb
1 avocado, peeled, stoned and
   cut into chunks
1 pear
juice of 1 lime
1 teaspoon fennel seeds
1 teaspoon cumin seeds
handful of mint leaves,
   finely chopped

Serves 2

This recipe was created out of love for the lonely fennel bulb that was staring at me from the fridge, saying, 'Eat me, I'm good for you!' I've learned, though, that fennel is something you either love or hate. It has an aniseed flavour that's quite bold. However, by mixing it with something sweet, like pear, and something a bit spicy, like the chilli flakes (red pepper flakes), the strong taste of the fennel is muted and complemented.

Preheat the oven to 180°C/350°F/gas 4 and line a baking sheet with parchment paper.

Coat the almonds in 1 teaspoon of the coconut oil, sprinkle with the cayenne pepper and spread out on the baking sheet. Toast for 10 minutes or until lightly browned.

Use a mandolin (or sharp knife) to slice the fennel thinly. Place in a medium bowl or on a large plate with the avocado. Peel the pear and grate it over the fennel and avocado, then squeeze over the lime juice to keep the pear from browning. Add the remaining coconut oil to a pan over a medium heat and toast the fennel and cumin seeds for 3 minutes. Toss the toasted seeds, almonds and mint over the salad and enjoy!

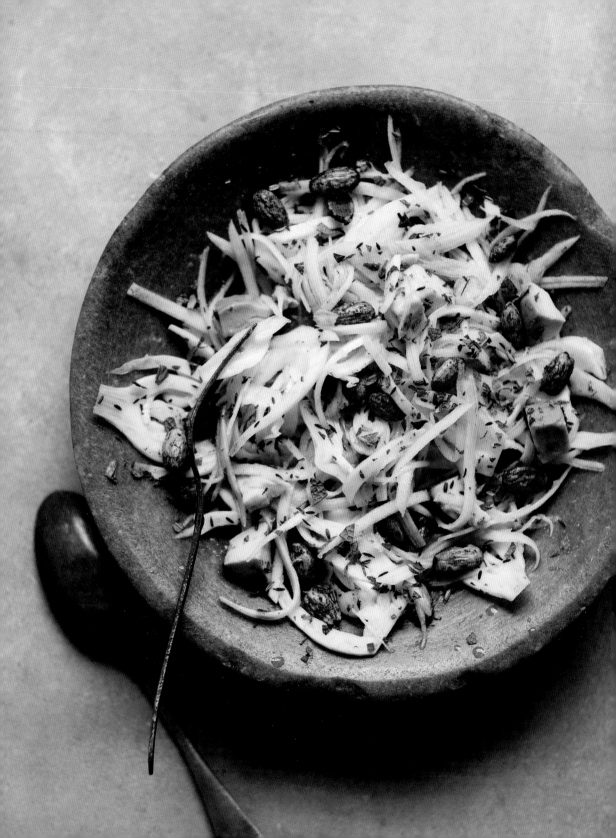

Burnt Corn, Kale and Lime Salad

2 corn cobs
1 teaspoon smoked paprika
1 teaspoon ground cumin
250g (6 cups) kale, shredded
approx.1 teaspoon sea salt
1 avocado, peeled, stoned and
   cut into small chunks

For the Dressing
handful of coriander (cilantro),
   torn
good squeeze of honey
juice of 1 lime

Serves 2

Creating delicious variations on the traditional side salad is something that I love to do. This recipe requires minimal preparation and can be put together in the 10 minutes before you serve your main meal. Kale is an ingredient that I tend to use a lot at home because of its amazing nutritional value. Adding lime juice to the salad dressing helps bring out the flavour of the other ingredients.

Using a sharp knife, cut the corn away from the cobs and separate into kernels. In a dry frying pan, cook the corn with the paprika and cumin for 10 minutes or until the corn starts to blacken. Remove the pan from the heat and allow to cool.

In a large bowl, massage the kale with the sea salt for 10 minutes or until it becomes soft. Whisk together the dressing ingredients in a separate bowl. Combine the burnt corn, avocado and kale, drizzle with the dressing, toss well and serve!

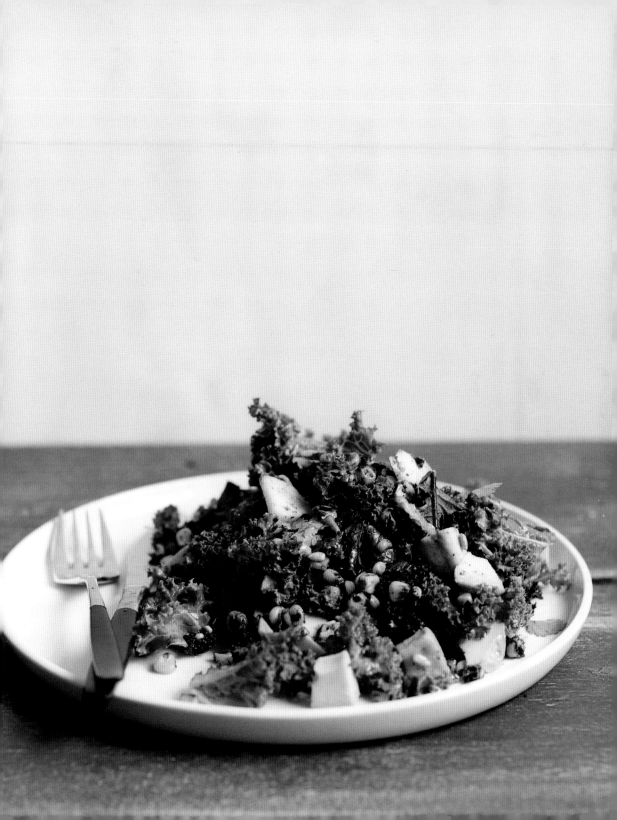

Beans, Beetroot and Herbs

8 cooked beetroot (beets) (very easy to find in your local supermarket), quartered
1 x 400g tin (1⅔ cups) white beans
small handful of pine nuts, toasted if preferred

For the Dressing
1 tomato
1 garlic clove
handful each of mixed mint, parsley and basil, plus extra, chopped, for garnishing
2 tablespoons capers
1 tablespoon olive oil
juice of 1 lemon
sea salt and freshly ground black pepper

Serves 2–3

This colourful dish can either be used as a very light lunch option or alternatively as a fantastic side dish. Beetroot (beets) are among the healthiest foods in the world and they contain a unique type of phytonutrient known as betalain. Research has shown that betalains are amazing for providing antioxidant, detoxification and anti-inflammatory support for the body. So you are eating an all-round winner!

Combine the beetroot and white beans in a large salad bowl. Blend all the ingredients for the dressing in a food processor or blender and use to coat the beetroot and beans.

Before serving, garnish with extra mint, parsley and basil as desired, and don't forget to top with your pine nuts. Enjoy!

Photographed with Lemon Lentil Salad with Peas, Radish and Dill (see page 52).

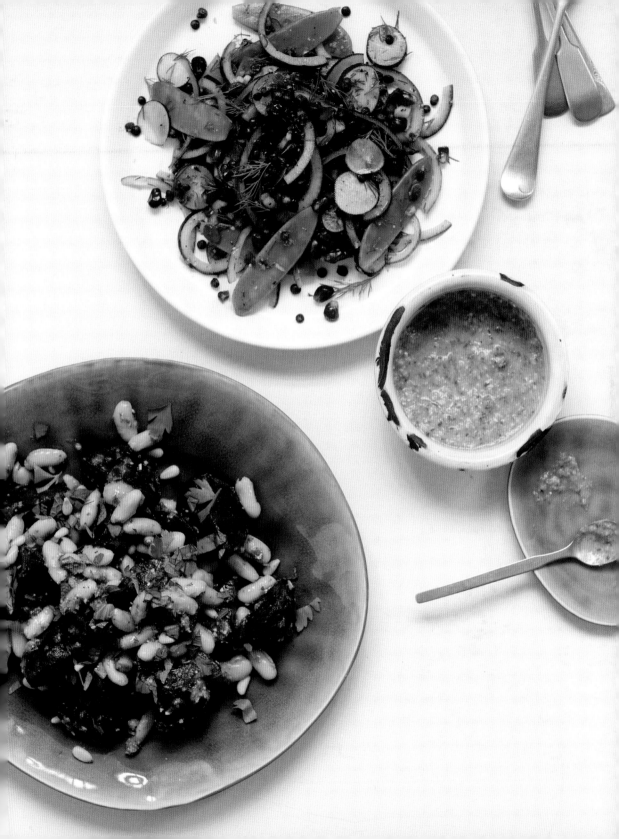

Lemon Lentil Salad
with Peas, Radish and Dill

150g (large handful)
  mangetout (snow peas)
1 x 400g tin (14oz) cooked Puy
  lentils, drained and rinsed
10 radishes, thinly sliced
large handful of dill, chopped
1 red onion, thinly sliced into
  half moons
large handful of pumpkin
  seeds
seeds from 1 pomegranate
1 avocado, peeled, stoned and
  chopped, optional
fresh greens, optional

For the Dressing
1 garlic clove, crushed
1 teaspoon wholegrain
  mustard
juice of 2 lemons
good squeeze of honey
sea salt and freshly ground
  black pepper

Serves 4

When it comes to easy recipes that pack a nutritional punch, lentils are my favourites. They are quick to make, taste yummy and are filled with all things good. With the addition of the peas, this is a very filling salad that's super easy to take out on the go. And the lemon dressing... well, it's to die for!

In a large bowl, combine the mangetout, lentils, radishes, dill, red onion, pumpkin seeds, pomegranate seeds and avocado, if using. And of course, feel free to add some fresh greens, too!

Whisk all the dressing ingredients in a small bowl, drizzle over the lentil mixture and toss to combine.

Photographed on page 51.

Smoked Paprika, Black Beans and Sprouting Broccoli Salad

250g (9oz) purple sprouting broccoli
1 x 400g tin (1⅔ cups) black beans, drained and rinsed
1 teaspoon smoked paprika
½ teaspoon ground cumin
1 tablespoon honey
2 spring onions (scallions), finely diced
1 avocado, peeled, stoned and cut into small chunks

For the Dressing
handful of coriander (cilantro)
small handful of blanched almonds, ideally soaked for a few hours, but don't worry if not!
2 tablespoons almond milk
juice of 1 lime

Serves 2

Purple sprouting broccoli brings an amazing combination of colour and crunch to a dish and is also, of course, rammed full of nutrients. The high vitamin and mineral content of broccoli, coupled with its exciting antioxidant count, make it an all-round winner for your health.

Bring a large pot of water to the boil and cook the broccoli for 5 minutes. Be careful not to overcook it so that you don't lose too many of the nutrients. Drain and rinse.

In a frying pan over a medium heat, combine the black beans, smoked paprika, cumin and honey. Stir this together well and cook for 5 minutes.

In a large bowl, combine the sprouting broccoli, seasoned black beans, spring onions and avocado. Finally, blend all the dressing ingredients in a food processor or blender until you have a lovely chunky dressing (that tastes great, too!) with which you can coat the broccoli and bean salad really well.

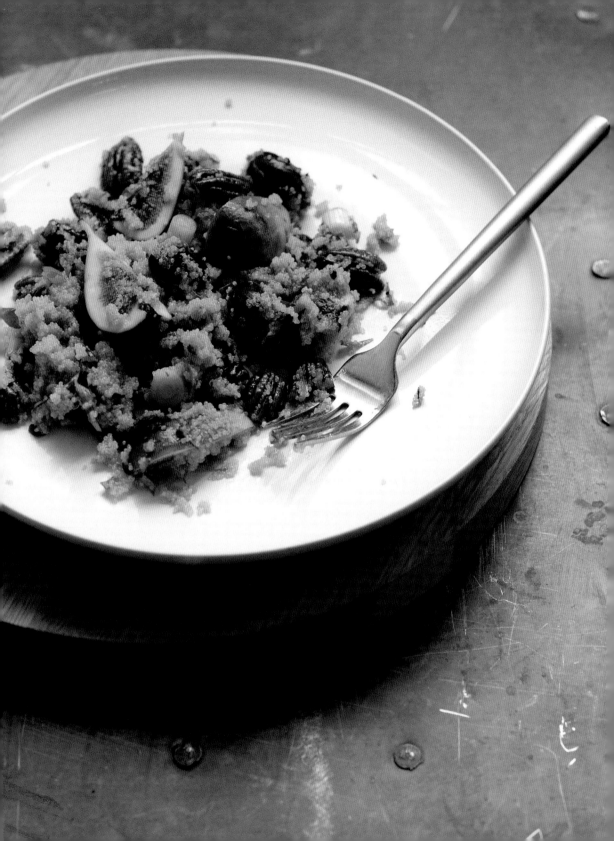

Amaranth, Olive and Fig Salad

200g (1 cup) uncooked
  amaranth
190g (1 cup) pitted black and
  kalamata olives
75g (⅔ cup) pecans
4 spring onions (scallions),
  chopped
½ teaspoon chilli flakes
  (red pepper flakes)
good squeeze of honey
juice of ½ lime, or to taste
4 fresh figs, quartered
4 tablespoons olive oil
handful of flat-leaf parsley,
  chopped
sea salt and freshly ground
  black pepper

**Serves 2–4 (depending how
  hungry you are!)**

For me, this is a kind of 'everything' salad. It's got your whole grain, your good fats, some dark greens and a bit of natural sweetness. So when you feel like you just need a good dose of as many nutrients as possible, let this be your go-to salad. And, luckily, it's easy, too!

Boil 600ml (2½ cups) water in a pan and add the amaranth. Cover and bring back to the boil, then reduce to a simmer for 15 minutes. Once cooked, drain off any excess water.

Meanwhile, place the olives, pecans, spring onions, chilli flakes, honey, lime juice and figs in a bowl and mix with the olive oil. Add the cooked amaranth and chopped parsley and mix well to combine. Add more lime juice if needed and season with sea salt and black pepper.

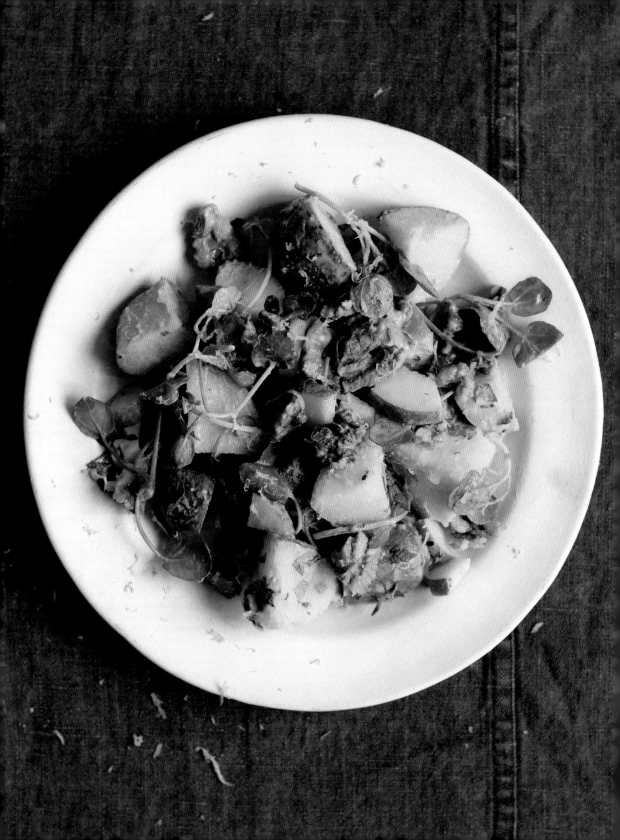

Immunity-boosting Red Potato Salad with Honey Tahini Dressing

6 red potatoes, quartered
  (keep the skin on!)
4 small handfuls of watercress
1 pear, cored and diced (keep
  the skin on!)
large handful of walnut halves,
  roughly chopped
small handful of mint, chopped
zest of 1 lemon
sea salt and freshly ground
  black pepper

For the Dressing
2 tablespoons tahini
2 tablespoons honey
juice of 1 lemon
2 tablespoons olive oil
1 teaspoon chilli flakes
  (red pepper flakes)

Serves 4

On those days when you might need to give your body a bit of a rest, such as after an indulgent weekend, this is the salad that will help support your liver and make you feel better and brighter in no time. The flesh of red potatoes is jam-packed with vitamin C – 45% of our RDA (recommended daily allowance) – and the skin provides most of the fibre. Not only does vitamin C boost immunity, it helps repair the body, too.

Put the potatoes into a large saucepan and cover with water. Bring to the boil over a high heat and cook until soft, about 15 minutes. Remove from the heat, drain and rinse with cool water.

Meanwhile, mix together the dressing ingredients in a small bowl and put to one side.

In a large bowl, combine the watercress, pear, walnuts and mint. Add the cooked red potatoes and coat with the honey and tahini dressing. Mix well, season with salt and pepper, garnish with the lemon zest and boom, your immune system will LOVE you!

Beetroot Noodle Salad with Clementine and Pistachios

2 good-sized beetroot (beets), peeled and spiralized
olive or coconut oil, melted, for drizzling
2 clementines, peeled and segmented
50g (heaping ⅓ cup) pistachios
2 tablespoons honey
2 large handfuls of fresh spinach
sea salt and freshly ground black pepper

For the Dressing
1 tablespoon olive oil
1 tablespoon apple cider vinegar
1 teaspoon wholegrain mustard
juice of 1 clementine
juice of ½ lemon

spiralizer

Serves 2

I know the latest craze is all about spiralized courgettes (zucchini) and trust me, I love them, too. But I wanted to experiment with other veggies that can give you the same lovely noodle shape, taste good and still deliver that nutritional punch. And so this is where the beetroot became my new courgette. But again, if you don't have beetroot to hand, please use a courgette instead!

Preheat the oven to 180°C/350°F/gas 4 and line 2 baking sheets with parchment paper. Place the beet noodles on one sheet and drizzle with olive or coconut oil. Season with salt and pepper and roast for 15 minutes.

Spread the clementine segments and pistachios over the second sheet and drizzle with the honey. Bake for 5 minutes alongside the beet noodles.

Meanwhile, whisk all the dressing ingredients in a small bowl and put to one side.

Once cooked, remove the baking sheets from the oven and combine the noodles, spinach, clementines and pistachios in a large bowl. Toss with the dressing and enjoy your simple but super-yummy salad!

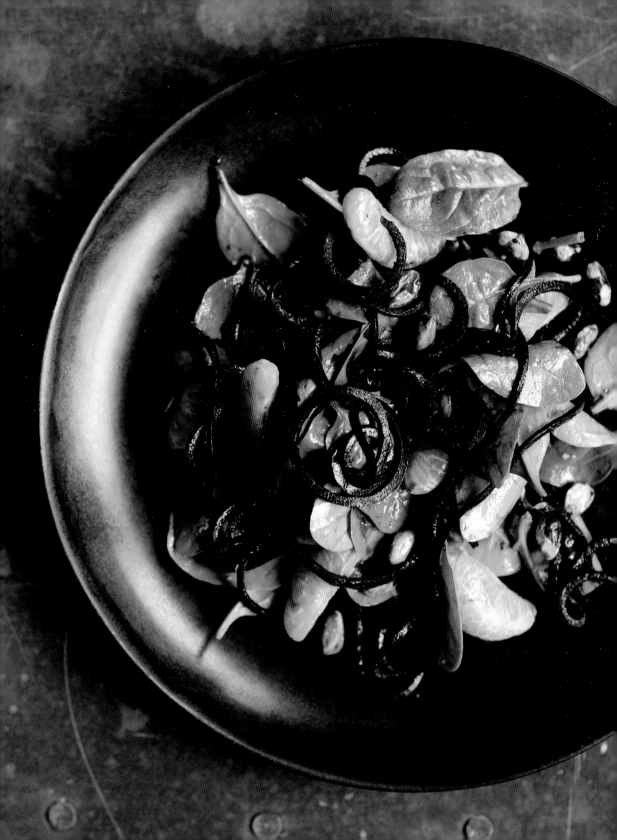

The Greenest Salad, Like Ever!

50g (heaping ⅓ cup) walnut halves
2 super-large handfuls of Brussels sprouts – about 12 – trimmed and shredded or finely grated
1 large bunch of kale, stems removed and leaves thinly sliced
handful of mint, chopped
1 green apple, cored and chopped

For the Dressing
1 small garlic clove, crushed
2 tablespoons olive oil
2 tablespoons apple cider vinegar
1 tablespoon Dijon mustard
1 teaspoon chia seeds, optional
juice of 1 lemon

Serves 2

Okay, so you say you don't like Brussels sprouts? I dare you to try to this salad and then let me know if you still don't like them! I grew up not wanting to see or eat Brussels sprouts, but then I discovered how good they are for me. These little guys are bursting with protein, fibre, vitamins, minerals and antioxidants. In fact, there's been a renewed interest in the emerging health benefits of Brussels sprouts recently. To be continued… But, for now, let's eat!

Preheat the oven to 180°C/350°F/gas 4 and place the walnut halves on a baking sheet. Bake for 10 minutes until lightly toasted.

Meanwhile, combine the Brussels sprouts, kale, mint and apple in a large bowl. In a separate small bowl, whisk together all the dressing ingredients.

Once the walnuts are toasted, mix into the salad and drizzle the dressing over the top. Toss well to combine and enjoy those Brussels sprouts and the Greenest Salad ever!

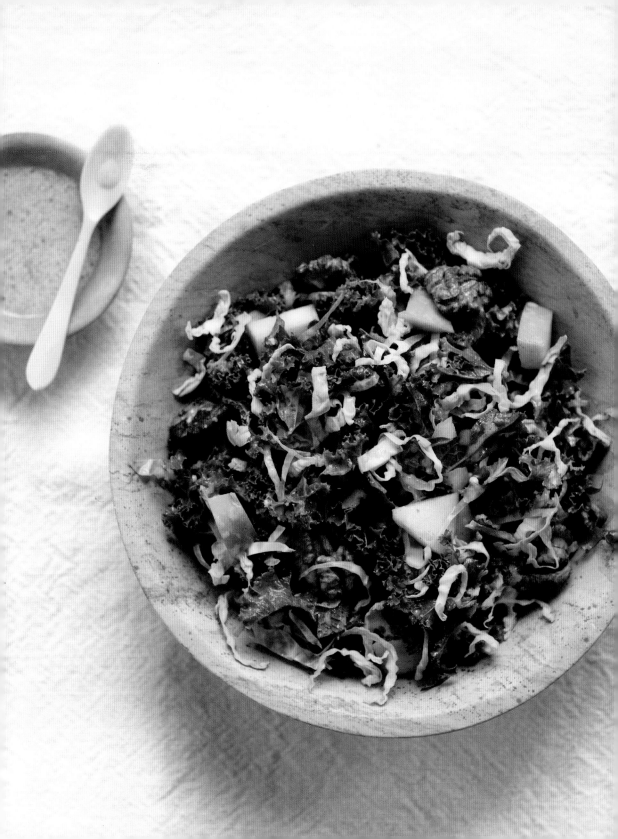

Spicy Red Cabbage Salad

I've previously struggled to get red cabbage into my diet. Red cabbage is some serious brain food. It's packed with vitamin K and anthocyanins that help with mental clarity. But these nutrients also improve your defence again dementia and even Alzheimer's. This is a super on-the-go salad that I love to eat once a week.

1 small red cabbage, finely shredded
1 x 200g tin (heaping ¾ cup) black beans, drained and rinsed
handful of coriander (cilantro), chopped
1 red (bell) pepper, seeds removed and chopped
½ cucumber, chopped
1 avocado, peeled, stoned and chopped
25g (3 tablespoons) sunflower seeds
2 tablespoons olive oil
juice of 1 lime
1 teaspoon chilli flakes (red pepper flakes)

Serves 2

Place the shredded cabbage in a large bowl with the black beans, coriander, red pepper, cucumber, avocado and sunflower seeds and mix well. In a small bowl, mix together the olive oil, lime juice and chilli flakes and drizzle over the cabbage salad.

And there you have it – an easy and delicious way to get that all-important red cabbage into your diet more regularly!

Photographed with Carrot Coleslaw Salad with Grapes (see page 64).

Jemima's Asian Slaw Salad

This comes from my lovely sister-in-law, Jemima. And I love how this recipe can be so much more than 'just a salad'. This is her take on it: "This is a wonderful accompaniment to any summer meal, and is especially great with grilled salmon. You can add shredded cooked salmon or chicken for a more filling mixture. We also love it rolled into fresh, crunchy spring rolls, dipped into a bit of homemade sweet chilli sauce." Even her two young children aged three and five love it, too! For me, that says it all... get cooking!

½ small white (green) cabbage (or ¼ large one), finely shredded
4 carrots, grated
2.5-cm (1-inch) piece fresh ginger, peeled and grated
1 cucumber, cut into thin strips or matchsticks
1 red chilli (chile pepper), seeds removed if you like, sliced into fine rings
zest and juice of 2 limes
2 tablespoons sesame seeds, toasted
sprinkle of coconut palm sugar
pinch of sea salt
handful of coriander (cilantro) leaves, chopped

Serves 4

Place the cabbage, carrots and ginger in a bowl with the cucumber, chilli and lime zest and juice and toss to combine. Add the toasted sesame seeds, toss again and add the sugar and salt as desired, plus the chopped coriander leaves.

Fresh, zingy and full of raw foods!

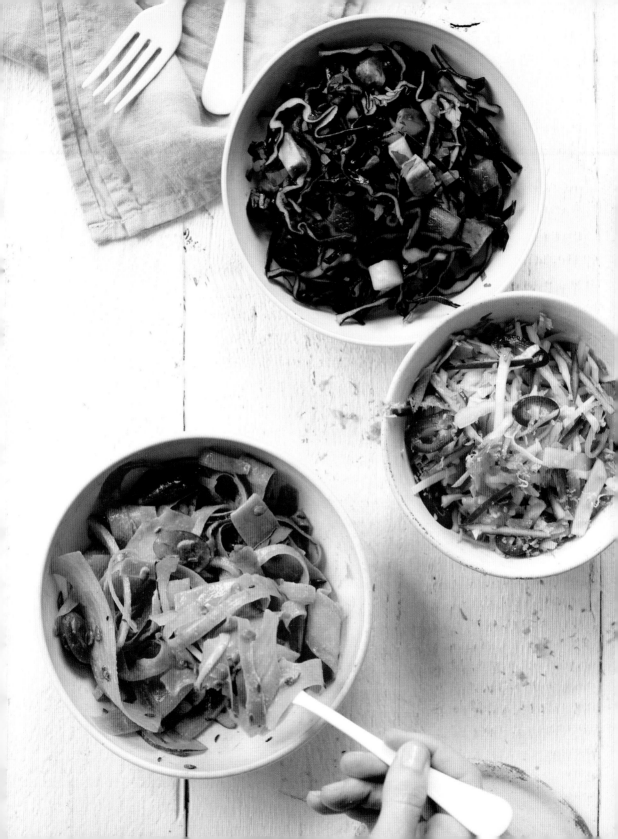

Carrot Coleslaw Salad with Grapes

4–6 carrots, peeled
12 red grapes, halved
½ red onion, thinly sliced
¼ teaspoon caraway seeds
40g (heaping ¼ cup) sunflower
  seeds (toasted, if preferred)

For the Dressing
1 garlic clove, crushed
50ml (3½ tablespoons) pure
  apple juice
2 tablespoons tahini
2 tablespoons honey
1 tablespoon apple cider
  vinegar
2 teaspoons curry powder

spiralizer or mandolin

Serves 2

In the past, I usually used carrots in a supporting role in my recipes, but I wanted to find one where they played the starring role, and this is it! You know the saying, 'An apple a day keeps the doctor away'? Well, I'm pretty certain the same applies to carrots, as they are filled with an abundance of must-have nutrients. This is an excellent way to get them in (and it tastes pretty darn good, too!).

If you have a spiralizer, then great – go at it and spiralize those carrots into thin strips. If you don't, don't worry! Use a mandolin to slice the carrots into wide strips. Place them in a large bowl with the grapes, red onion, caraway seeds and sunflower seeds.

In a separate small bowl, whisk together the dressing ingredients until smooth. Thoroughly mix the dressing into the carrot strips so that they are very much coated with the dressing. Wait about 5 minutes to allow the dressing to really soak into the carrots and then devour!

Photographed on page 63.

Mexican Corn Salad
with the Best Herb Dressing

4 corn cobs
large handful of coriander
  (cilantro), chopped
1 small red onion, finely diced
1 red chilli (chile pepper),
  seeds removed and finely
  chopped
1 large tomato, chopped
coconut oil, for rubbing

For the Dressing
½ ripe avocado, peeled
1 garlic clove, crushed
small handful of coriander
  (cilantro)
1 tablespoon olive oil
¼ teaspoon chilli (chili) powder
zest and juice of 1 lime

Serves 4

I wrote about corn in my first book, *Superfoods*, because I grew up in the middle of Illinois cornfields. I love this stuff so much. Yet another thing I miss from back home is Mexican food. I mean, c'mon, they know how to mix their spices up! So, this salad combines my love of corn with my love of Mexican food, making it a perfect addition to those Mexican-inspired meals.

Preheat a large griddle (grill) pan over a medium-high heat. Rub the corn with some coconut oil and grill each cob until the kernels are lightly charred, about 5 minutes, turning occasionally. Remove from the heat and allow to cool.

Meanwhile, blend together all the dressing ingredients in a food processor or blender until smooth. If the dressing is too thick for your liking, add a couple of tablespoons of water.

Now, back to the corn! Using a sharp knife, slice the corn kernels from the cob, then transfer them to a large bowl. Add the chopped coriander, red onion, chilli and tomato, drizzle over the dressing and toss to combine.

This salad can be served immediately, while the corn is still warm, or make it ahead and eat it later.

Butternut Squash and Sweet Potato Salad

2 small sweet potatoes, peeled
  and cubed
½ butternut squash, peeled,
  seeds removed and cubed
coconut oil, melted, for rubbing
2 spring onions (scallions),
  thinly sliced on the diagonal
4 radishes, thinly sliced,
  optional

For the Dressing
120ml (½ cup) coconut or soya
  yogurt
1 tablespoon apple cider
  vinegar, or more if preferred
1 teaspoon wholegrain
  mustard
1 garlic clove, crushed
small handful of coriander
  (cilantro), chopped
sea salt and freshly ground
  black pepper

Serves 4

This is a great twist on an oldie but goodie – the traditional potato salad. The great thing about this salad is that it's brightly coloured, which means that it's packed with antioxidants and loads of other good-for-your-body nutrients. Remember, a good rule to follow is that the darker the colour of your fruit or vegetable, the more of a specific nutrient will be found in that food.

Preheat the oven to 200°C/400°F/gas 6 and line a baking sheet with parchment paper. Tip the sweet potato and butternut squash chunks onto the sheet and massage them with a good amount of coconut oil so that the cubes are covered in the oil. Roast on your middle shelf for 15 minutes, or until just tender.

Meanwhile, whisk together the dressing ingredients in a large bowl. Add a bit more vinegar if you prefer a thinner dressing.

Once the squash and potatoes are cooked, add them to the bowl and coat thoroughly with the yogurt dressing. Top with the sliced spring onions and radishes, if using.

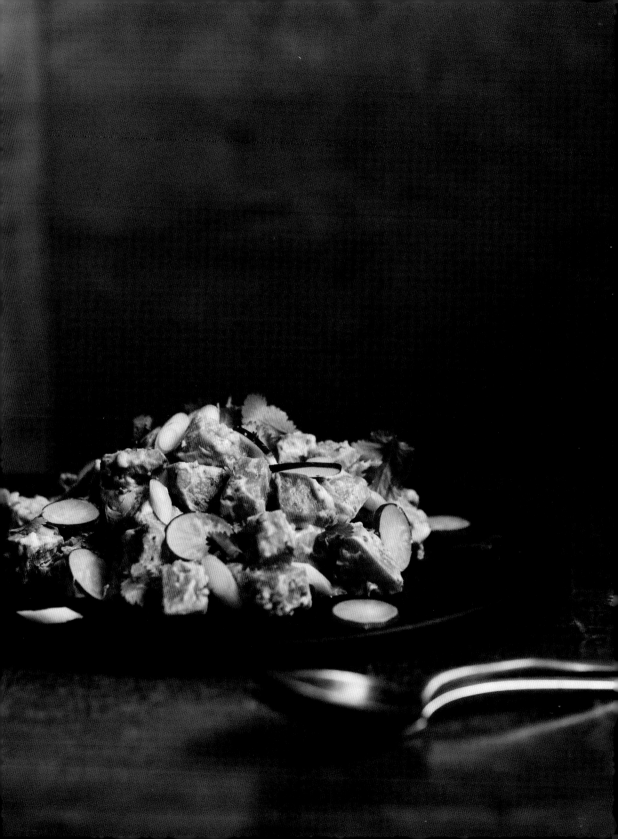

Garlic Spinach Salad with Roasted Butter Beans

1 x 400g tin (1⅓ cups) butter (lima) beans, drained and rinsed
2 tablespoons olive oil, plus extra for drizzling
2 tablespoons ground cumin
250g (5½ cups) fresh spinach
good handful of pine nuts

For the Dressing
1 whole head of garlic, cloves separated but skins on
2 tablespoons tahini
2 tablespoons honey or maple syrup
1 tablespoon olive oil
1 tablespoon apple cider vinegar
1 teaspoon wholegrain mustard
juice of 2 lemons

Serves 2–3

I love making roasted chickpeas (garbanzo beans) for a snack or to add to pretty much any salad or soup. However, I decided to go against the grain for this recipe and roast butter (lima) beans instead. Absolutely delicious! And that's the thing about beans: as long as they are hearty enough, roast away. Oh, and P.S., if you love garlic, then you'll love this dressing, but perhaps make sure you eat it on a non-date night!

Preheat the oven to 200°C/400°F/gas 6 and line a baking sheet with parchment paper.

Put the beans into a mixing bowl and toss with the olive oil and cumin. Spread them out on the baking sheet with the garlic cloves for the dressing and drizzle with just a bit more olive oil. Bake for 10–12 minutes until lightly browned, then remove from the oven to cool for a couple of minutes.

Squeeze the garlic out of the skins into a food processor or blender with the remaining dressing ingredients and blend. Put the spinach into a large bowl and coat it thoroughly with the garlic dressing. Sprinkle over the pine nuts and butter beans, then thoroughly enjoy!

Millet Cashew Salad with Mango Dressing

1 tablespoon olive oil
1 teaspoon cumin seeds
juice of 1 lemon
200g (1 cup) uncooked millet
75g (⅔ cup) cashews
small handful of parsley,
   chopped

For the Dressing
1 large ripe mango, peeled,
   stoned and roughly chopped
1 garlic clove, crushed
1-cm (½-inch) piece fresh
   ginger, peeled and grated
small handful of coriander
   (cilantro)
juice of ½ lime
sea salt and freshly ground
   black pepper

Serve 4

Millet is a super-easy grain to cook in less than 20 minutes AND you're getting a surge of energy that will last for several hours. So, for me this is a great salad to eat on those day when you have a long time before your next meal – maybe a long meeting to attend or a long flight – when this salad will keep you full and satisfied for hours.

Pour 480ml (2 cups) water into a large saucepan over a medium-high heat. Add the olive oil, cumin seeds, lemon juice and millet and bring to the boil, stirring a couple of times to stop the millet sticking to the pan. Then reduce the heat to low, cover and simmer for 18–20 minutes until the liquid has been absorbed and the millet is fluffy.

Meanwhile, blend the dressing ingredients in a food processor or blender.

Once the millet is cooked, place in a large bowl, add the cashews and parsley and drizzle the mango dressing over the top before mixing well. Enjoy your energy extender!

Braised Cauliflower Couscous with Orange Tofu

200g (1¼ cups) uncooked wholewheat giant couscous
400ml (1¾ cups) boiling water or vegetable stock
2 tablespoons coconut oil, plus extra if needed
1 small cauliflower, cut into small florets and even use the stalks!
1 teaspoon sweet paprika
1 teaspoon ground cinnamon
250g (9oz) firm tofu, drained and crumbled
zest and juice of ½ orange
1 tablespoon honey
1 tablespoon nutritional yeast
small handful of mint, finely chopped
2 spring onions (scallions), sliced
good handful of flaked (slivered) almonds
sea salt and freshly ground black pepper

Serves 4

I think I've saved the best for last in the Super Salads section. You've got to be quick with this one to get it into 20 minutes, but moving from one thing to another makes it so much fun, and trust me, it's delicious. I always look for ways to spice up my tofu, and the orange in this recipe really works well with all the ingredients. I hope you enjoy this real Super Salad!

Place the couscous in a large bowl (this will be the main bowl, so make sure it's big enough) and cover with the boiling water or veggie stock. Cover and leave until the liquid is absorbed.

Melt the coconut oil in a large frying pan over a medium-high heat. Add the cauliflower and cook, stirring regularly, for 10 minutes. Sprinkle the cauliflower with the paprika and cinnamon and continue to cook for another 2 minutes, making sure the cauliflower is nicely coated. Remove from the heat and add to the couscous.

Add the crumbled tofu to the same pan (feel free to add a bit more coconut oil) and cook until slightly golden, about 3 minutes. Add the orange zest and juice, honey and nutritional yeast and coat the tofu well. Fry for another minute, then add to the couscous. Mix the salad well and gently stir in the mint, spring onions and flaked almonds. Season to taste.

And that, my friends, is a super-gorgeous salad to be devoured immediately!

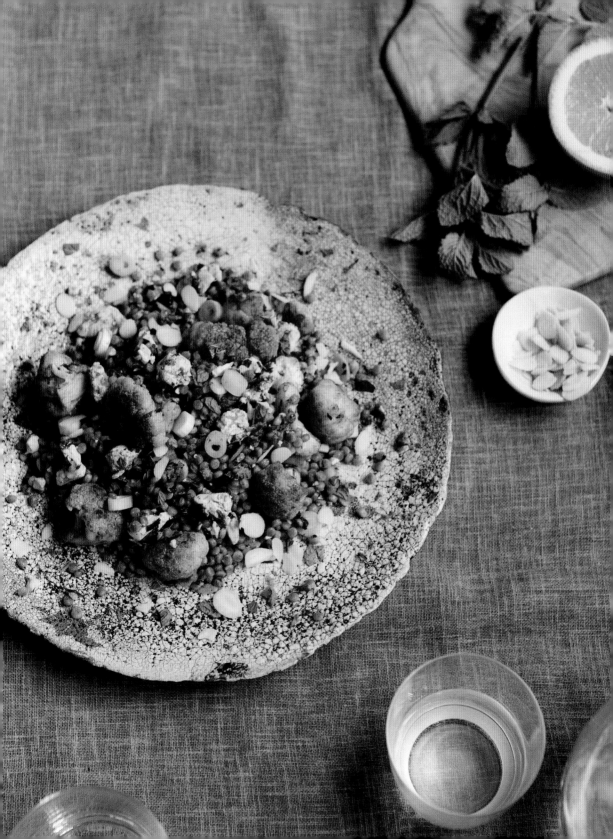

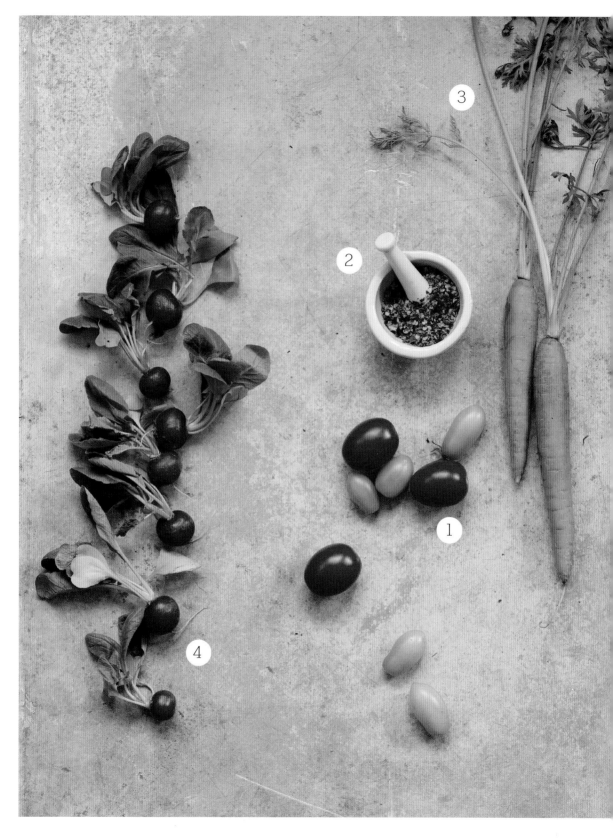

super SOUPS

Soups do the body good, they really do. They are so warming and soothing, that sometimes I almost feel like someone has just given me a big hug after eating a bowl! P.S. These soups are great on their own or, for a bigger meal, serve them with your favourite toasted bread. (I'm a big fan of rye!)

superfood superheroes

1. Tomatoes
Tomatoes are incredibly nutrient dense and we could all surely benefit from including them in our diets more regularly! As well as providing the body with several of the essential vitamins and minerals that it needs, tomatoes also help to prevent chronic disease. This disease-fighting ability comes from the presence of lycopene, which is a phytonutrient that has particularly strong links to battling certain cancers.

2. Chilli flakes (red pepper flakes)
Chilli flakes get their taste and spicy kick from capsaicin, which is known to combat inflammation in the body as well as being heralded as a natural painkiller when applied topically. Consuming chilli flakes regularly is shown to lower blood cholesterol and they also act as a powerful natural decongestant.

3. Carrots
Carrots are a popular food and they provide several important health benefits. Not only do they contain high levels of fibre, vitamin K, potassium and beta-carotene, but they are also linked to weight loss, lowered cholesterol levels and improved vision.

4. Radishes
Radishes are cruciferous vegetables that have a unique flavour. Their crunchy texture makes them a pleasure to eat and they are amazing for soothing sore throats, aiding digestion and helping to prevent infection. Regular consumption of radishes is also thought to help rid the body of damaging toxins.

Roasted Tomato, Sweet Potato and Chia Soup

3 large tomatoes, halved
olive oil, for drizzling
2 sweet potatoes, peeled and
  chopped
400ml (1¾ cups) vegetable
  stock
2 tablespoons honey
handful of coriander (cilantro),
  leaves picked and torn,
  to garnish
1 tablespoon chia seeds,
  for sprinkling
2 spring onions (scallions),
  thinly sliced

Serves 2

Sweet potatoes are inexpensive, delicious and readily available all year round. They are also a great source of magnesium, which is the relaxation and anti-stress mineral. So whip up a batch of this for those nights when you need to sleep well.

Preheat the oven to 220°C/425°F/gas 7. Place the tomato halves on a baking sheet, drizzle with olive oil and roast for 10 minutes.

While the tomatoes are roasting, boil the sweet potatoes for 10 minutes in a large saucepan of boiling water, then remove, drain and rinse. Tip the drained potatoes back into the pan with the vegetable stock, lower the heat and leave to simmer.

Remove the roasted tomatoes from the oven and add them to the pan along with the honey before blitzing with a stick blender.

Serve in bowls, garnished with the torn coriander leaves and sprinkled with the chia seeds and the sliced spring onions.

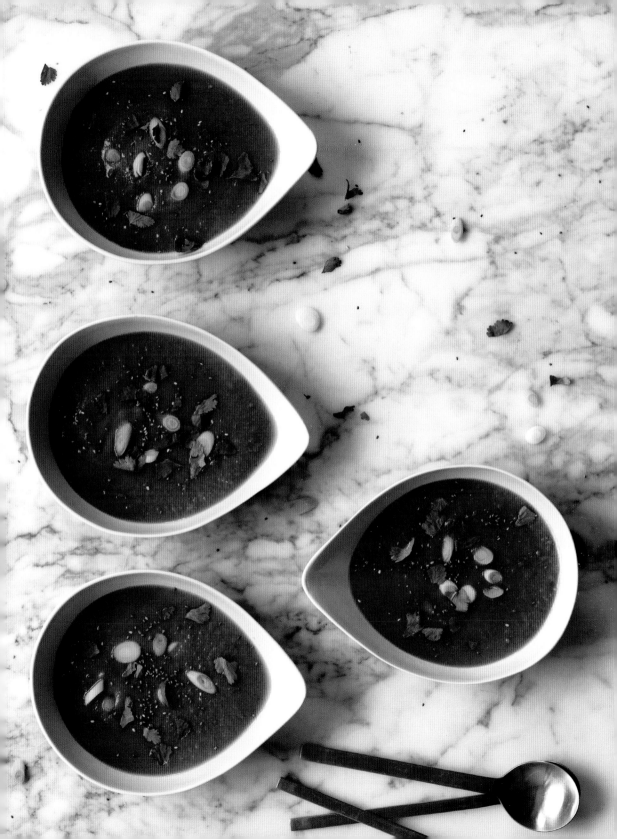

Creamy Courgette and Sage Soup

1 tablespoon coconut oil
3 celery sticks, finely chopped
2 medium courgettes
  (zucchini), chopped
10–12 radishes, chopped
200ml (¾ cup + 1½ tablespoons)
  vegetable stock
200ml (¾ cup + 1½ tablespoons)
  coconut milk
1 teaspoon dried sage
1 teaspoon cayenne pepper
fresh sage leaves, finely sliced,
  to garnish, optional

Serves 2

Courgettes (zucchini) are incredibly low in calories and the fibre in the skin helps burn fat, so if you are looking to have a bowl of 'low-cal' 'detox' soup, then this recipe is your new best friend.

First, melt the coconut oil in a large saucepan over a medium heat. Add the chopped celery, courgettes and radishes and fry for 5 minutes. Next, add the vegetable stock and coconut milk, simmering over a medium-high heat for 10 minutes. Add the dried sage and cayenne pepper and stir for 3 more minutes.

Either whizz to a purée in a food processor or blender, or serve straightaway and garnish with finely sliced fresh sage, if using.

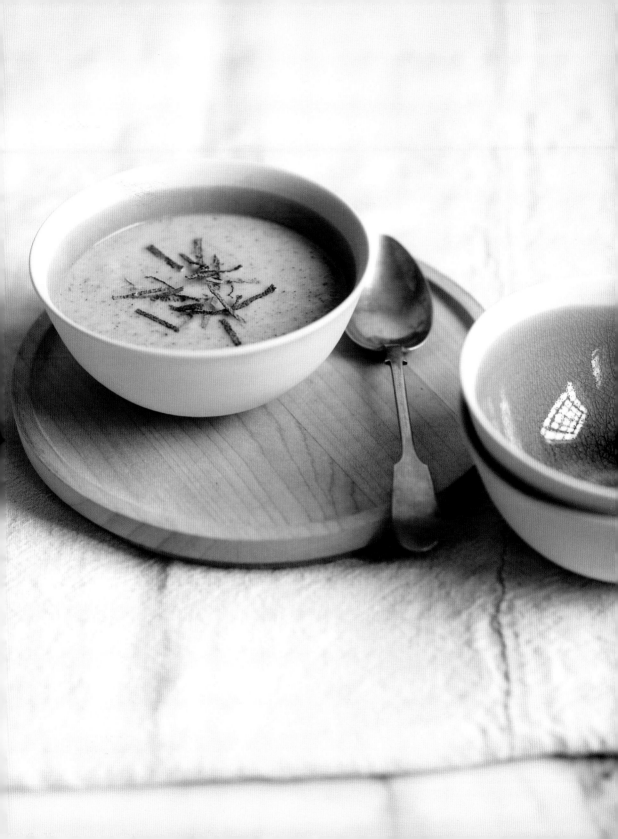

Warming Broccoli and Tofu Soup

1 tablespoon coconut oil
2 celery sticks, chopped
1 medium onion, diced
1 teaspoon apple cider vinegar
500g (4 cups) broccoli florets
200ml (¾ cup + 1½ tablespoons)
  vegetable stock
150g (5½ oz) silken (soft) tofu
2 tablespoons pumpkin seeds,
  for sprinkling
sea salt and freshly ground
  black pepper

Serves 2

Believe it or not, broccoli contains high levels of calcium and vitamin K, both of which are important for healthy bones and osteoporosis prevention. So, eating broccoli throughout your entire life is a really good thing.

Melt the coconut oil in a heavy-based saucepan over a medium-high heat. Add the celery and onion and fry for 3 minutes. Season with salt and pepper and then add the cider vinegar. Add the broccoli to the pan and cover with just enough boiling water to submerge the florets. Stir in the vegetable stock and leave to simmer for 5 minutes.

Once the broccoli has cooked through, put the whole mixture into a food processor or blender. Add the tofu and blend until completely smooth. Return to the pan to reheat, adjusting the seasoning as necessary.

Serve in deep bowls, sprinkled with the pumpkin seeds.

Photographed with Chunky Tomato Soup (see page 80).

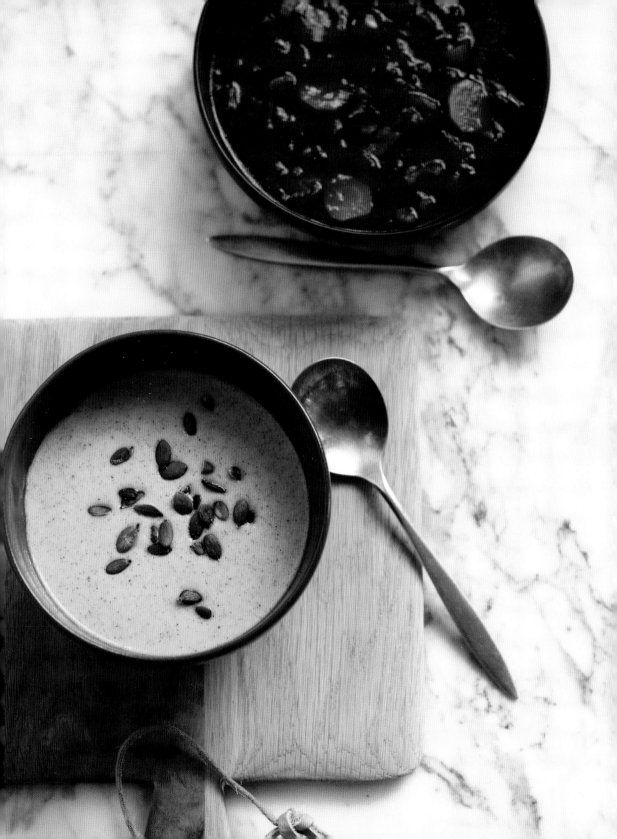

Chunky Tomato Soup

2 x 400g tins (3½ cups) chopped
  tomatoes
2 celery sticks, chopped
150g (1 cup) cherry tomatoes
2 carrots, sliced
200ml (¾ cup + 1½ tablespoons)
  vegetable stock
large handful of basil, chopped
2 tablespoons honey
sea salt and freshly ground
  black pepper

Serves 2–3

The lycopene in tomatoes is a natural antioxidant
that works to slow the growth of cancerous cells. And
guess what – cooked tomatoes produce even more
lycopene than their raw counterparts. So go ahead
and keep cooking that tomato soup!

Add the chopped tomatoes, celery, cherry tomatoes
and carrots to a large saucepan over a medium-high
heat and stir for a few minutes before adding the
vegetable stock. Continue to cook and stir occasionally
for 10 more minutes, lowering the heat after 5 minutes.

Stir in the basil and honey, heat for a few more minutes
and then serve in bowls, seasoned with salt and
pepper to taste.

Photographed on page 79.

Simple Minestrone with Fresh Spinach

1 x 400g tin (1¾ cups) chopped tomatoes
400ml (1¾ cups) vegetable stock
1 x 400g tin (1⅓ cups) cannellini beans, drained and rinsed
1 x 200g tin (1 cup) kidney beans, drained and rinsed
50g (scant 1 cup) fresh spinach
sea salt and freshly ground black pepper

Serves 2

Spinach is one of the most nutritious vegetables around. It's not only high in vitamins and minerals, but also in phytonutrients, which act as powerful antioxidants to help protect our cells and DNA.

Add the chopped tomatoes to a large saucepan over a medium heat and simmer for a few minutes before adding the vegetable stock and all the beans. Continue to cook for 7–8 minutes before lowering the heat and adding the spinach leaves.

Stir for a few more minutes before serving in bowls and seasoning with salt and pepper.

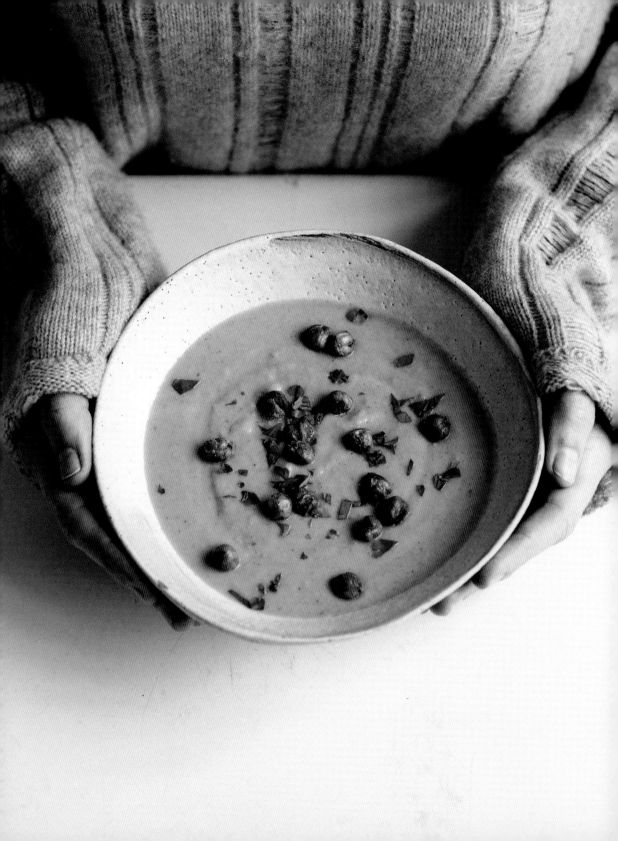

Spicy Carrot and Chickpea Soup

1 tablespoon coconut oil
5 carrots, sliced
400ml (1¾ cups) coconut milk
200ml (¾ cup + 1½ tablespoons)
  vegetable stock
1 teaspoon ground cumin
1 x 400g tin (1½ cups) chickpeas
  (garbanzo beans), drained
  and rinsed
2 teaspoons chilli flakes
  (red pepper flakes)
small handful of flat-leaf
  parsley, chopped, to garnish
Crunchy Cumin Chickpeas
  (see page 30), to garnish,
  optional

Serves 2

The doctor was right: carrots are good for your eyesight. They won't cure pre-existing problems, but they can protect against sight problems caused by a deficiency in vitamin A. And so this is a super-simple soup for those nights when you just can't be bothered to really cook… But the good news is that it sure is good for you.

Melt the coconut oil in a large saucepan over a medium-high heat. Add the carrots and cook for 3 minutes. Pour in the coconut milk and vegetable stock along with the cumin and stir well.

Continue to cook for 10 minutes before adding the drained chickpeas. Lower the heat and stir well before mixing in the chilli flakes. Stir for a few more minutes and then whizz to a purée in a food processor or blender.

Serve in bowls, garnished with the parsley and your Crunchy Cumin Chickpeas, if using.

Broccoli and Butter Bean Soup with Flaxseed

1 tablespoon coconut oil
2 garlic cloves, minced
1 small onion, diced
150g (3 cups) chopped broccoli
1 x 400g tin (1⅓ cups) butter (lima) beans, drained and rinsed
400ml (1¾ cups) vegetable stock
1 teaspoon paprika
1 tablespoon flaxseed (linseed), to garnish

Serves 2

Looking for protein without the fat? Well, butter (lima) beans are a wonderful source of protein – yes protein! And considering they are low in fat, butter beans are a super-healthy alternative to fatty meats that are actually high in cholesterol and saturated fat.

Melt the coconut oil in a frying pan over a medium-high heat. Add the garlic, onion and broccoli and fry for 3–5 minutes until softened and browned.

Meanwhile, add the butter beans to a large saucepan along with the vegetable stock and simmer over a medium-high heat. After a few minutes, add the browned broccoli, onion and garlic and continue to simmer for 10 minutes.

Remove the pan from the heat, add the paprika and blitz with a stick blender. Serve in bowls and garnish with the flaxseed.

Red Lentil and Sweetcorn Soup

120g (¾ cup) sweetcorn (corn)
400ml (1¾ cups) vegetable
  stock
100g (½ cup + 1 tablespoon)
  uncooked split red lentils
1 x 400g tin (1¾ cups) chopped
  tomatoes
1 red onion, diced
1 teaspoon chilli flakes
  (red pepper flakes)
handful of coriander (cilantro)

Serves 2

Sweetcorn (corn) is a rich source of antioxidants, which fight cancer-causing free radicals. And unlike many other foods, cooking corn actually increases the amount of usable antioxidants, just like tomatoes.

Preheat the oven to 220°C/425°F/gas 7 and line a baking sheet with foil or a silicone mat. Spread out the sweetcorn on the foil or mat and bake for 10 minutes.

Meanwhile, add the vegetable stock and lentils to a large saucepan over a medium-high heat and leave to simmer for 5 minutes. Add the chopped tomatoes and onion to the pan and cook for a further 5 minutes before blitzing with a stick blender. Lower the heat and continue to simmer as you stir in the chilli flakes.

Serve in bowls sprinkled with the baked sweetcorn and garnished with the coriander.

Speedy 'Pot Noodle' Soup

500ml (2 cups + 2 tablespoons)
  vegetable stock
2.5-cm (1-inch) piece fresh
  ginger, peeled and minced
1 garlic clove, minced
150g (5½ oz) uncooked soba
  noodles
60g (1 cup) fresh beansprouts,
  plus a few extra to garnish
60g (small handful) mangetout
  (snow peas), chopped
juice of 1 lime
1 teaspoon chilli flakes
  (red pepper flakes)
sea salt and freshly ground
  black pepper
zest of 1 lime, to garnish,
  optional

Serves 2

For those of you who just might be addicted to Pot Noodles, this is your healthy answer and it's almost just as quick to make! Its lovely thick texture makes this a super-hearty meal, plus mangetout contains 128% of the recommended daily allowance of vitamin C per cup. Vitamin C is a powerful antioxidant that helps the body develop resistance against infection.

Bring the vegetable stock, ginger and garlic to the boil in a large saucepan over a medium-high heat before adding the noodles and lowering the heat to a simmer. Stir the noodles and then add in the beansprouts and mangetout. Continue to stir until you can see that the noodles are thoroughly cooked. Squeeze in the lime juice and chilli flakes and season to taste.

Stir again before removing from the heat and serving in bowls, garnished with a few more beansprouts and lime zest, if using.

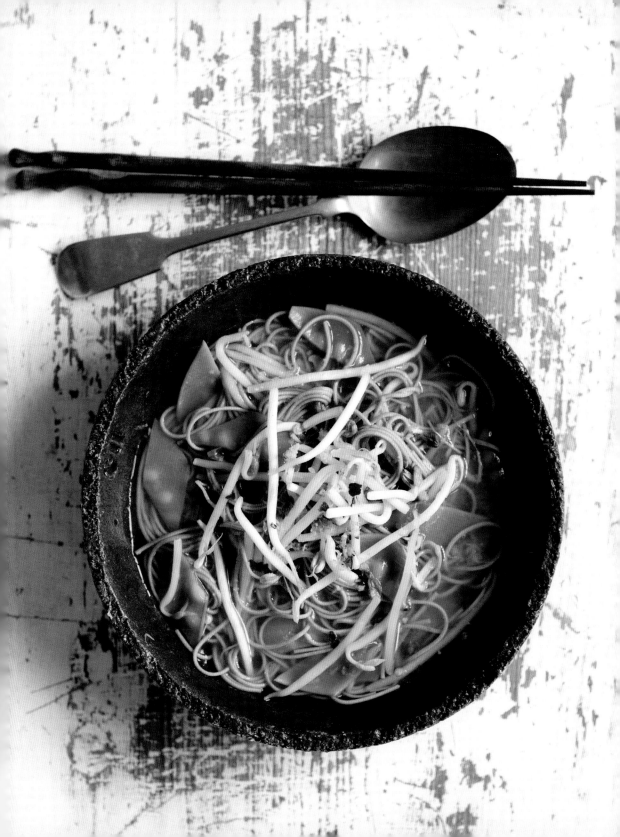

Avocado Gazpacho

600g (3 cups) tinned plum
  tomatoes, roughly chopped
½ cucumber, peeled and
  roughly chopped
½ red (bell) pepper, chopped
1 avocado, peeled and stoned
1 teaspoon lemon juice
½ teaspoon apple cider
  vinegar
1 garlic clove, roughly
  chopped
1 tablespoon olive oil
1 teaspoon chilli flakes
  (red pepper flakes)
sea salt and freshly ground
  black pepper

Serves 2–4

Avocados contain more potassium than bananas and 77% of the calories from avocado are from fat. Yes, it is one of the fattiest foods on the planet! However, this isn't just any fat, this is oleic acid, a monounsaturated fatty acid that has been linked to reduced inflammation in the body and is considered a 'heart-healthy' fatty acid.

Put all the ingredients, except for half the avocado, the olive oil and the chilli flakes, in a food processor or blender with 40ml (2½ tablespoons) water. Blend until fairly smooth and then add the olive oil. Blend again until smooth, tasting to check the seasoning.

Serve in bowls with the remaining avocado chopped and sprinkled on top, or in slices on the side, with the chilli flakes.

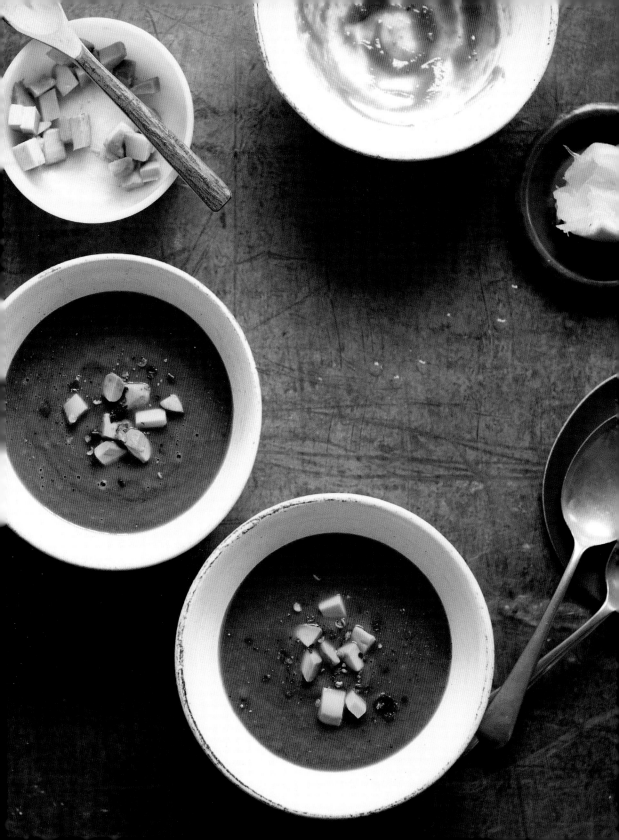

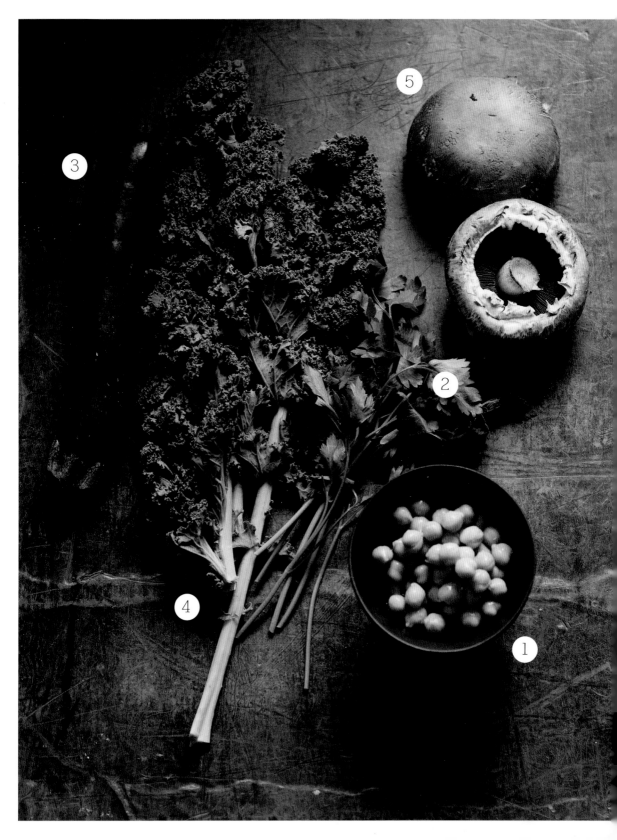

super SQUARE MEALS

I think the French got it right with this one. Lunch should be your biggest meal of the day. I mean, think about it, it's right in the middle of the day and you still have the rest of your afternoon to get through, and the early evening. If you're anything like me, I eat lunch around 12.30pm and supper around 7pm – that's a long time between your meals. Yes, of course you can have some healthy snacks in between, but we want that lunch to go as far as it can before we reach for them. So, I've created these lunches with the 'square meal'– a substantial, satisfying, and balanced meal – in mind. Go get 'em, tiger!

superfood superheroes

1. Chickpeas (Garbanzo beans)
Chickpeas are incredibly high in nutrients and can easily be added into your regular diet. They are low in fat but high in fibre, making them great for digestion as well as helping you to feel full for longer. They also contain a wealth of protein, which makes them a fantastic plant-based source of this essential compound.

2. Parsley
Parsley is one of the most popular herbs in the world and with good reason! There are two very unusual components found within it: the first is a selection of oil components and the second is a range of flavonoids. These elements work to promote optimum health as well as inhibiting the development of certain cancers.

3. Courgette (Zucchini)
Courgettes boast an impressive nutritional profile due to the range of phytonutrients, vitamins and minerals found in them. They are an especially great source of vitamin C and manganese, which means consuming courgettes regularly can help to protect against tissue damage. Regular consumption will also help your body metabolize cholesterol.

4. Kale
Kale is among the most nutrient-dense foods in existence and you can actually hit several of your daily nutrient quotas with just one cup of raw kale! This one cup will contain more than 100% of your recommended daily allowance of vitamins A, C and K. It also contains impressive amounts of vitamin B6, manganese, calcium, copper, potassium and magnesium.

5. Mushrooms
Mushrooms often taste better when cooked but are healthiest in their raw form. Whichever way you decide to prepare them, they will still provide some fantastic health benefits. Mushrooms contain selenium, which is great for the function of the bladder and the thyroid. They are low in calories while providing a healthy dose of vitamin D and iron.

Fried Brown Rice with Tofu and Peanut Sauce

180g (1 cup) uncooked brown
  rice
250g (9oz) firm tofu
1 tablespoon coconut oil
1-cm (½-inch) piece fresh
  ginger, peeled and grated
2 red chillies (chile peppers),
  thinly sliced
2 garlic cloves, crushed
1 red onion
1 carrot, sliced
2 tablespoons peanut butter
2 tablespoons tamari
1 tablespoon honey (or other
  natural sweetener)
1 spring onion (scallion), sliced
  on the diagonal, to garnish

Serves 2

Brown rice is actually quick to cook as long as you keep it slightly boiling. And I love adding brown rice to any meal because, for me, it makes it more substantial and keeps my energy levels at the perfect point over the next several hours. This lunch is also easy to whip up, put in an airtight container and take away with you wherever you're bound.

Preheat the oven to 180°C/350°F/gas 4 and line a baking sheet with parchment paper. Bring a pan of water to the boil and add the rice as soon as it hits boiling point, then turn down the heat just very slightly so that the water is still lightly boiling and leave to cook for 15 minutes.

Drain the excess water from the tofu by pressing it between paper towels with your hands, then cut into small chunks, transfer to the prepared baking sheet and bake for 10 minutes.

Meanwhile, heat the coconut oil in a large frying pan and add the ginger, red chillies and the garlic. Give the pan a stir while you chop the red onion and then add that into the mix. When the onion starts to brown, add the carrot slices and cook for 2–3 minutes.

Next, mix together the peanut butter, tamari and honey in a bowl. If you prefer a thinner sauce you can stir in 2 tablespoons water. Continue to stir the pan for a few more minutes, then drain the brown rice and add it to the pan with the baked tofu. Mix well and then pour the sauce on top as you continue to stir.

Serve in bowls, garnished with the sliced onion.

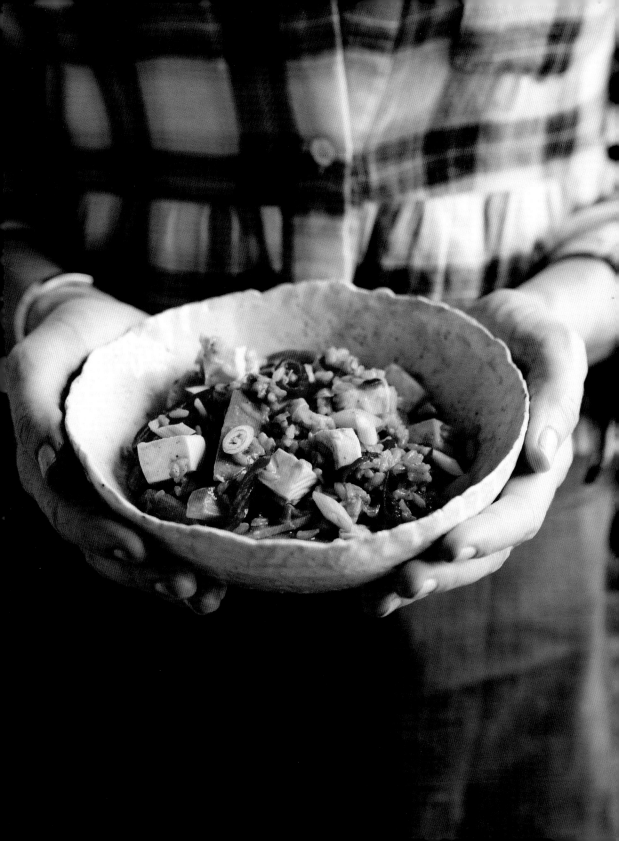

Sweet Potato and Spinach Bowl

1 large sweet potato, peeled
 and cut into chunks
1 tablespoon coconut oil
90g (1¾ cups) broccoli florets
1 onion, diced
1 x 400g tin (1⅔ cups) black
 beans, drained and rinsed
120g (¾ cup) sweetcorn (corn)
6 cherry tomatoes
1 teaspoon ground cumin
handful of fresh spinach
olive oil, for drizzling

Serves 2

When you want a quick meal, this is the way to go.
I love this bowl because it's also very pretty. It's a
rainbow of different colours, and as we know, it's a
good thing when we eat a rainbow of different foods.

Bring a medium pan of water to the boil and add the
sweet potato chunks.

Meanwhile, heat the coconut oil in a frying pan and
fry the broccoli with the onion and the black beans,
cooking for a few minutes, stirring occasionally. Add
the sweetcorn and cherry tomatoes before sprinkling
the cumin on top.

Continue cooking both pans for a further 5 minutes and
then drain the sweet potato and add it to the pan with
the broccoli. Stir together and then serve in bowls with
the spinach on top, drizzled with olive oil.

Curried Couscous

Curry isn't just for supper. I can seriously have a curry any time of the day – well, maybe not for breakfast, but definitely for lunch that's for sure. So, this recipe is a wonderful lunch curry using wholewheat giant couscous (my favourite) instead of rice and it's absolutely delicious and filling.

1 tablespoon coconut oil
½ medium onion, diced
1 carrot, sliced
2 tablespoons green curry paste
½ teaspoon ground turmeric
½ teaspoon paprika
400ml (1¾ cups) coconut milk
200ml (¾ cup + 1½ tablespoons) vegetable stock
185g (1¼ cups) uncooked wholewheat giant couscous
1 x 400g tin (1½ cups) chickpeas (garbanzo beans), drained and rinsed
juice of ½ lime
handful of coriander (cilantro)

Serves 2

Heat the coconut oil in a large saucepan over a medium heat and add the onion and carrot. Stir for a moment and then add the green curry paste, turmeric and paprika and stir for 2 minutes. Pour in the coconut milk and the vegetable stock and continue to stir.

Next, add in the giant couscous and the chickpeas and leave to simmer for 10 minutes. Once cooked, squeeze over the lime juice and garnish with the coriander.

Farro and Chickpea Stew

Farro is fast gaining attention as the new super 'grain' on the block becuase of its nutritional punch. A very similar texture to rice, farro is a great source of protein, fibre and iron. Make no mistake, this ancient grain is set to make a huge comeback.

300g (2 cups) cherry tomatoes, halved
3 garlic cloves, minced
1 small onion, diced
100g (½ cup) farro
1 x 400g tin (1½ cups) chickpeas (garbanzo beans), drained and rinsed
large handful of rocket (aragula)
large handful of fresh spinach
handful of basil
sea salt
coconut oil, melted, for roasting

Serves 2

Preheat the oven to 200°C/400°F/gas 6 and line a baking sheet with parchment paper. Place the tomatoes, garlic and onion on the baking sheet and drizzle some coconut oil over the top. Roast for 15 minutes.

Meanwhile, bring a pan of water to the boil, add the farro and cook a few minutes, then reduce the heat to a simmer and leave to cook for 15 minutes. Remove from the heat and drain away any excess water, then tip the chickpeas into the pan and stir well to combine. Add in the rocket and spinach and stir again.

Serve the farro mixture on plates, topped with the baked tomatoes, garlic and onion, garnished with the basil and seasoned with a sprinkling of salt.

Tostadas with Herb Hummus

For the Hummus
1 x 400g tin (1½ cups) chickpeas
  (garbanzo beans), drained
  and rinsed
1 garlic clove, chopped
handful of parsley
handful of dill
handful of coriander (cilantro)
2–3 tablespoons olive oil
2 tablespoons tahini
pinch of sea salt

For the Salsa
2 tomatoes
1 red onion
1 red chilli (chile pepper)
handful of coriander (cilantro),
  chopped
juice of ½ lime

For the Tostadas
200g (1½ cups) sweetcorn (corn)
4 corn tortillas
olive oil, for brushing
1 avocado, peeled, stoned and
  chopped
3 jalapeño peppers, sliced

Serves 2

This recipe pretty much just requires a food processor or blender. It's about tossing good ingredients in and combining them with other delicious flavours to make a perfectly blended lunch. There are days when I just love whoever invented the food processor!

Preheat the oven to 220°C/425°F/gas 7 and line a baking sheet with parchment paper. Place the sweetcorn for the tostadas on the sheet and bake for 10 minutes.

Meanwhile, make the hummus by blending all the ingredients in a food processor or blender. Next, transfer to a bowl and then blend all the salsa ingredients very briefly just to roughly chop them. Once complete, transfer the salsa to another bowl and place in the fridge with the hummus while you prepare the tostadas.

Start by brushing a little olive oil on each corn tortilla and then place them in the preheated oven alongside the sweetcorn. After 5–10 minutes the tostadas will turn crispy and you can then remove them from the oven with the sweetcorn.

Place the tostadas on plates with a spoonful of hummus, avocado, jalapeños and sweetcorn on each one. The salsa can be served on top or on the side for dipping.

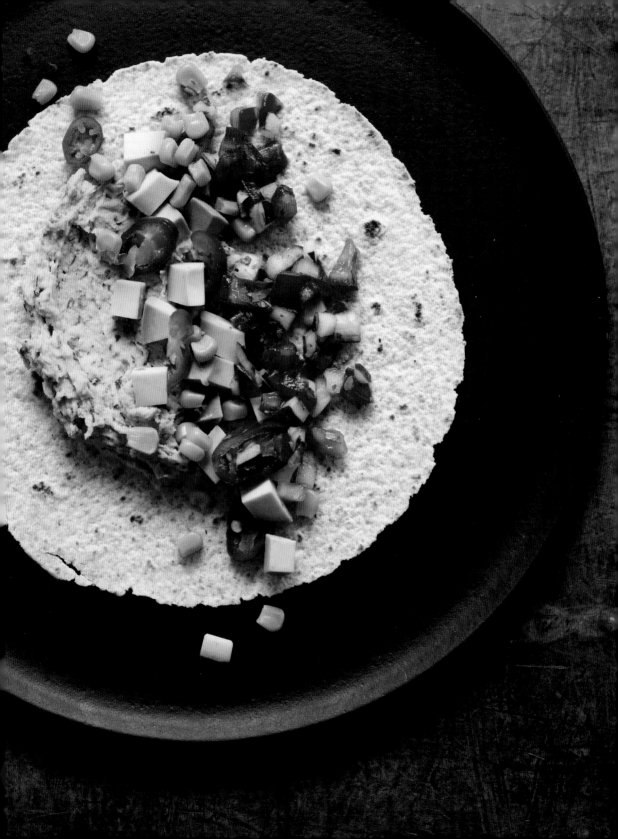

Tofu and Kale Scramble

1 tablespoon coconut oil
½ red onion, diced
250g (9oz) firm tofu, drained
  and crumbled
½ teaspoon ground turmeric
150g (4 cups) kale
100g (¾ cup) pitted olives,
  sliced
sea salt and freshly ground
  black pepper
sliced avocado and/or cherry
  tomatoes, to serve, optional

Serves 2

Growing up I definitely had my fair share of scrambled eggs for lunch and this, for me, is just a better version of it, especially with the kale and turmeric – my favourite green and my favourite spice. For a heartier lunch, add a corn tortilla for your 'bread/grain' option.

Heat the coconut oil in a frying pan and cook the onion until it begins to brown. Add the tofu to the pan and use a spatula to mash it until it is broken down well, then add the turmeric. Continue to stir as you add the kale. Once the kale begins to wilt, add the olives.

Mix everything together well and season with salt and pepper before serving, topped with sliced avocado and cherry tomatoes, if using.

Lunch in a Jar

These recipes are true on-the-go Square Meals that you can take anywhere. I first thought about making a 'lunch in a jar' after seeing something similar at my local supermarket, but wowsers were they expensive! So these jars are my take on what I saw but, for me, healthier, more satisfying and definitely cheaper.

Spicy Noodle Jar

1 packet instant rice noodles
1 vegetable stock cube
80g (½ cup) cooked edamame beans
2 red chillies (chile peppers),
   finely sliced into rings
1 red (bell) pepper, seeds removed and
   chopped
120g (3 cups) kale
1 teaspoon ground ginger

2 Kilner/Mason jars, cleaned and dried

Serves 2

Divide the noodles between the jars. Place half the stock cube in each jar, followed by half each of the rest of the ingredients. Then simply add a cup of hot water to each jar when you are ready to eat, seal the lid and shake well to allow the stock cube to dissolve.

It's that easy!

Photographed on page 101.

Herbed Chickpea Jar

1 tablespoon coconut oil
2 x 400g tins (3 cups) chickpeas (garbanzo
   beans), drained and rinsed
1 teaspoon ground cumin
1 teaspoon dried coriander
1 teaspoon dried parsley
2 large handfuls of fresh spinach
olive oil, for drizzling
sea salt and freshly ground black pepper

2 Kilner/Mason jars, cleaned and dried

Serves 2

Heat the coconut oil in a frying pan over a medium-high heat and heat the chickpeas through for a few minutes, then sprinkle the cumin, coriander and parsley over the top. Stir well and continue to cook for a few more minutes.

Divide the spinach between the two jars, followed by 2 tablespoons of chickpeas for each one. Continue to layer in this way until all the chickpeas and spinach are used up. Drizzle olive oil over the top and season to taste.

Photographed on page 101.

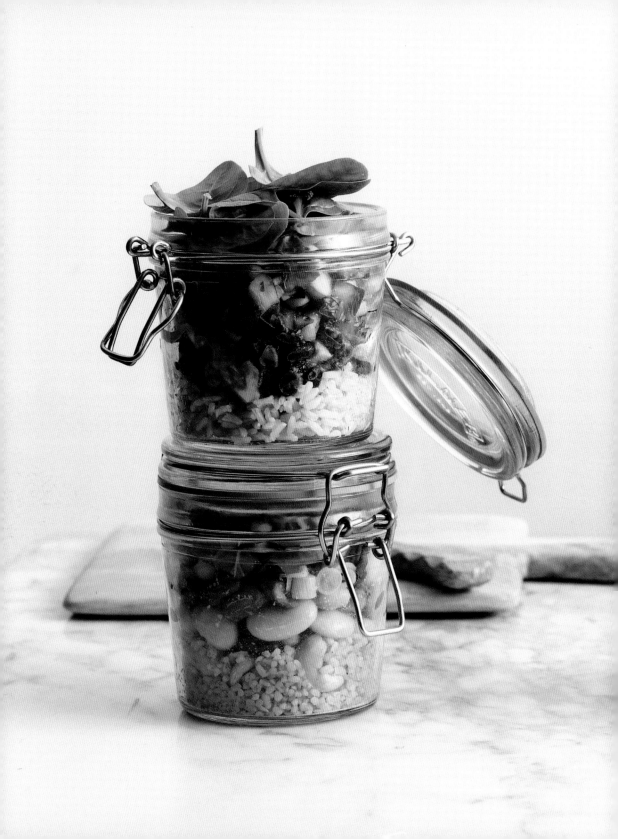

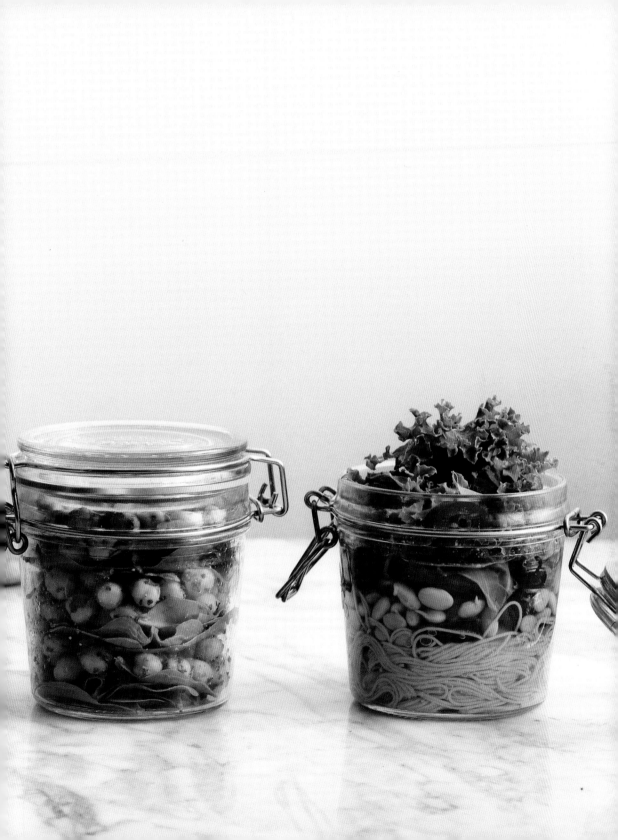

Burrito Salad Jar

Bulgur Wheat and Beans Jar

180g (1 cup) uncooked brown rice
2 tomatoes, chopped
1 red onion, diced
handful of coriander (cilantro), chopped
200g (1¼ cups) tinned black beans,
   drained and rinsed
½ avocado, peeled, stoned and chopped
juice of 1 lime
olive oil, for drizzling
handful of fresh spinach

2 Kilner/Mason jars, cleaned and dried

Serves 2

Cook the brown rice in boiling water over a medium-high heat for 15 minutes. Meanwhile, stir together the tomatoes, red onion and coriander in a bowl.

Place the black beans and avocado in a separate bowl and mix with the lime juice and olive oil. Mash everything with a fork for a few moments.

As soon as the rice is cooked, drain any excess water and allow it to cool for a moment before you spoon it into the jars. Top each portion with black bean mixture then tomato mixture. Place some spinach at the top of each jar and seal!

Photographed on page 100.

120g (¾ cup) uncooked bulgur wheat
2 tablespoons coconut oil
2 garlic cloves, minced
100g (¾ cup) tinned pinto beans
100g (⅔ cup) tinned butter (lima) beans
40g (⅓ cup) cashews
1 teaspoon ground cumin
1 teaspoon paprika
2 spring onions (scallions), chopped
handful of basil, chopped
sea salt and freshly ground black pepper

2 Kilner/Mason jars, cleaned and dried

Serves 2

Cook the bulgur wheat in boiling water over a medium heat for 10–12 minutes. Meanwhile, heat 1 tablespoon of the coconut oil in a frying pan over a medium-high heat and cook the garlic and all the beans for 10 minutes, stirring occasionally, then lower the heat to medium.

Drain the bulgur wheat if needed. Tip back into the pan, lower the heat and add the remaining coconut oil with the cashews and spices. Season, and stir for a few minutes. Spoon the bulgur mixture into the jars, then the bean mixture and the onions and basil.

Photographed on page 100.

Cannellini Bean Patties with Greens

1 x 400g tin (1⅓ cups) cannellini beans, drained and rinsed
½ courgette (zucchini)
3 tablespoons coconut oil
2 garlic cloves, finely chopped
2 spring onions (scallions), chopped
½ teaspoon apple cider vinegar
a few sprigs of fresh flat-leaf parsley, roughly chopped
½ tablespoon any wholegrain (whole-wheat) flour
3 tablespoons polenta
sea salt and freshly ground black pepper

For the Greens
Simple! Any greens you wish to include – but make sure you include some healthy superfoods!

Serves 2

I was so used to eating cannellini beans in salads all the time and I love them so much (they're possibly my top choice of bean), that I wanted to make them more than just a 'salad bean'. So I created this recipe to make the bean outshine the green – for once.

Place the beans in a bowl and season with salt and pepper. Gently mash the beans until the paste is fairly thick and dough-like. Take the courgette and grate it evenly into the bowl.

Heat a tablespoon of the coconut oil in a frying pan over a medium-high heat and fry the garlic and onions with the apple cider vinegar until the onions are soft, then tip the mixture into the bowl with the mashed beans. Mix well, checking the seasoning and adjusting to taste. Add the parsley, flour and 1 tablespoon of the polenta to the bowl. If your mixture is still sticking to the sides of the bowl, add a bit more polenta.

Separate the mixture into four and shape each one into patties – they should stay whole without cracking or falling apart. Coat the patties in the rest of the polenta, ensuring an even coverage.

Heat the rest of the coconut oil in a frying pan over a medium-high heat and fry the patties for 5 minutes on each side (you can make your salad while you wait!). When the patties are ready, they will be crunchy and golden brown – perfect for eating alongside your healthy greens!

Courgetti Spaghetti with Grapefruit and Brazil Nut Pesto

40g (⅓ cup) brazil nuts
¼ teaspoon sea salt
handful of basil
handful of coriander (cilantro)
2 tablespoons olive oil
1 garlic clove
juice of ½ lemon
2 medium courgettes
  (zucchini), spiralized
1 grapefruit, peeled and
  segmented

spiralizer

Serves 2

In the mood for a light summer salad? Well, lighter than pasta, courgette (zucchini) noodles check that box. Seasoned with a gorgeous – not your run-of-the-mill – pesto and topped with grapefruit, this salad might just be the envy of your co-workers!

Place the brazil nuts, salt, basil, coriander, olive oil and garlic in a food processor or blender with the lemon juice and 3 tablespoons water. Blend to make your pesto.

In a bowl, coat the courgette spaghetti with the pesto, then divide between bowls and top with the lovely grapefruit pieces!

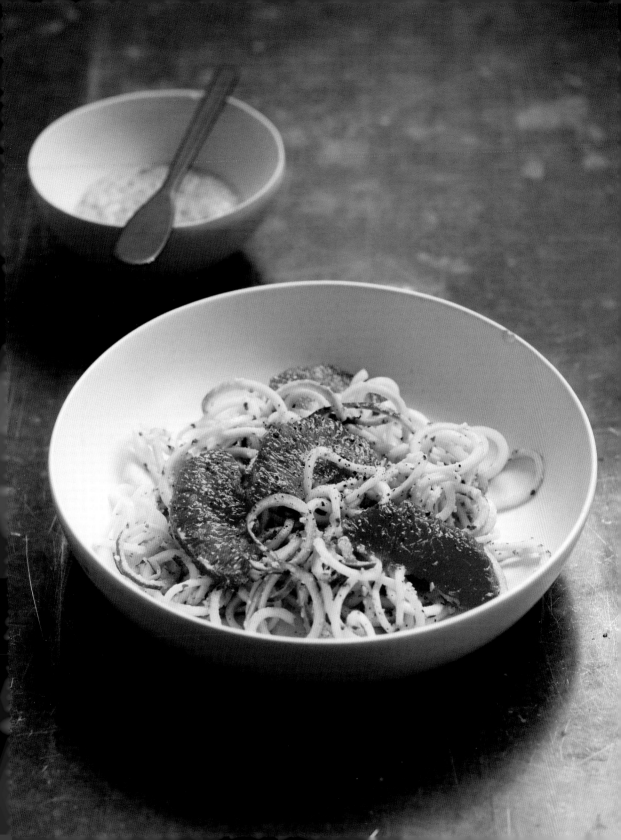

Curried Chickpeas with Cauliflower Rice

1 tablespoon coconut oil
1 x 400g tin (1½ cups) chickpeas (garbanzo beans), drained and rinsed
1 tablespoon curry powder
200ml (¾ cup + 1½ tablespoons) coconut milk
½ cauliflower head, cut into chunks
½ teaspoon ground cumin
handful of coriander (cilantro)
50g (1 scant cup) fresh spinach

Serves 2

I have recently become obsessed with cauliflower. And in particular, making cauliflower rice. I even spotted a bag of 'ready-made' cauliflower rice in a nearby supermarket! I'm not quite sure that cauliflower is the new 'kale' just yet, but it's certainly giving kale a run for its money with the amount of goodness each bite contains. This is a fun one.

Heat the coconut oil in a frying pan over a medium-high heat. Add the chickpeas and curry powder, stirring for a few moments, and then pour in the coconut milk. Lower the heat and leave to simmer while you make your cauliflower rice.

Place the cauliflower, cumin and coriander in a food processor and pulse until the cauliflower looks like rice, then remove and divide between bowls.

Stir the spinach into the chickpea mixture and leave to simmer for 2 minutes, then spoon it over the cauliflower rice. It's that simple... and fun!

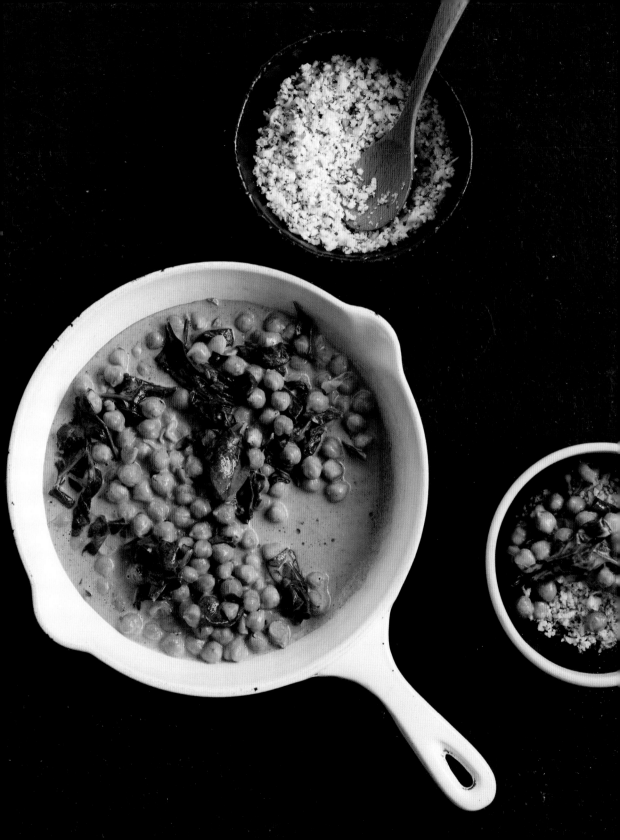

Tabbouleh with Edamame and Pomegranate

125g (¾ cup) uncooked bulgur wheat
1 tablespoon coconut oil
1 large tomato, chopped
1 small onion, diced
100g (1½ cups) button mushrooms, halved
large handful of flat-leaf parsley, finely chopped
2 tablespoons lemon juice
seeds of 1 pomegranate
50g (scant ½ cup) cashews, chopped
80g (½ cup) cooked edamame beans

Serves 2

This is my heartier take on traditional tabbouleh, to make it more of a meal than just a salad. I added a couple of my hero foods – mushrooms, edamame, pomegranate and cashews – to give this square meal more of a nutritional punch and a bit more colour, too.

Bring a pan of water to the boil and add in the bulgur wheat before lowering the heat and simmering for 15 minutes.

Meanwhile, heat the coconut oil in a frying pan and cook the tomato, onion and mushrooms over a low heat for 7–10 minutes.

Drain the cooked bulgur wheat, if necessary, and combine with the mushroom mixture in a large bowl together with the parsley, lemon juice, pomegranate seeds, cashews and edamame.

Mix together with a spoon and serve.

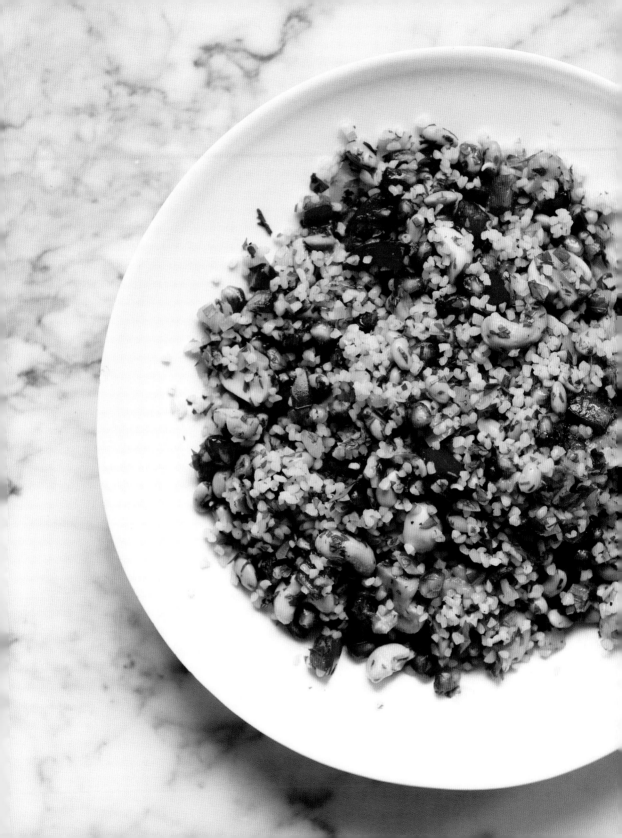

Tofu Skewers with Green Goddess Sauce

3 tablespoons coconut oil
150g (5½oz) extra-firm tofu, drained and patted dry with paper towels
1 red onion, cut into chunks
1 courgette (zucchini), cut into chunks
30g (½ cup) dried porcini mushrooms, cut into chunks and rehydrated according to manufacturer's instructions
1 red (bell) pepper, seeds removed and cut into chunks
sea salt and freshly ground black pepper

For the Sauce
½ large avocado, peeled
small handful of coriander (cilantro)
3 tablespoons olive oil
juice of 1 lemon
sea salt and freshly ground black pepper

skewers, soaked for 10 minutes in water if wooden

Serves 2

Perfect for a summer barbecue or easy enough to cook under the grill (broiler), especially if you're taking it 'to go'. The sauce is just super. Once again, you can use this sauce on so much more – roasted veg, salads fish… it's the perfect accompaniment to any meal in my view.

Blend all the sauce ingredients together in a food processor or blender, tasting to make sure the seasoning and lemon are to your taste. Pop in the fridge while you make the skewers.

Heat a barbecue or grill (broiler) to medium. Put the coconut oil in a medium frying pan and heat until hot, but not overly spitting. Fry the tofu for a few minutes until it is nearly golden brown, then remove it with a slotted spoon. Pour the melted coconut oil from the pan over the veggies in a bowl, tossing to coat.

Carefully skewer the veggies and tofu, season with salt and pepper and barbecue or grill for about 10 minutes, turning every 5 minutes so that they don't burn. When they're ready, serve with lashings of sauce on top.

Utterly delicious!

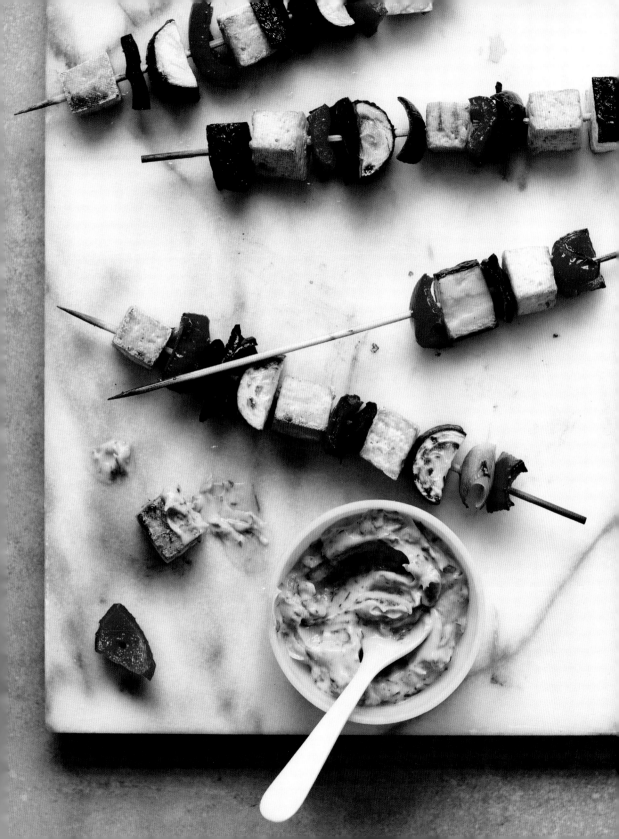

Baked Chickpeas and Kale

1 x 400g tin (1½ cups) chickpeas
  (garbanzo beans), drained,
  rinsed and patted dry with
  paper towels
½ tablespoon lemon zest
extra virgin olive oil,
  for coating
lemon juice, for drizzling
handful of pumpkin seeds
sea salt and freshly ground
  black pepper

For the Kale
240g (6 cups) kale
extra virgin olive oil
½ teaspoon garlic powder
pinch of sea salt

Serves 2

I eat a lot of chickpeas (garbanzo beans) for lunch because I find them very filling and obviously very good for me, too! I love this recipe not only because it's simple, but because it makes the chickpeas just a bit more interesting and, in my view, more tasty. Add some good fresh kale – or spinach is perfect; just get that green in – and you've got the ideal lunch to get you through your day.

Preheat the oven to 220°C/425°F/gas 7 and line 2 baking sheets with parchment paper.

Toss the chickpeas in the lemon zest and extra virgin olive oil and season with salt and pepper, then spread onto one of the lined baking sheets. Bake for 10 minutes.

Meanwhile, put the kale in a large mixing bowl along with the extra virgin olive oil, garlic powder and salt. Toss together until completely coated. Spread out the kale on the second baking sheet and put it in the oven with the chickpeas for another 5 minutes.

Remove both sheets from the oven and arrange on plates, drizzled with lemon juice and sprinkled with the pumpkin seeds.

Garlic and Agave Tofu Stir Fry

190g (1 cup) uncooked quinoa,
  well rinsed
150g (5½oz) firm tofu
1 tablespoon sesame oil
100g (1 cup) trimmed and
  chopped asparagus spears
1 carrot, sliced
2 spring onions (scallions),
  chopped
100g (2⅔ cups) kale, chopped

For the Sauce
1 garlic clove
1-cm (½-inch) piece fresh
  ginger
2 tablespoons agave nectar
2 tablespoons soy sauce
1 tablespoon sesame oil

Serves 2

I absolutely love this sauce. Not only is it great in this recipe, but it can be used on roasted vegetables, on any whole grain, over a piece of meat or fish and even as a salad dressing! Therefore, make sure you fold this page so that you always have it on hand whenever you need to spice up a dish.

Bring a pan of water to the boil over a medium-high heat and cook the quinoa – about 15 minutes, lowering the heat to a gentle simmer after 5 minutes.

Meanwhile, add all the sauce ingredients along with 1 tablespoon water to a food processor or blender and blitz until smooth. Next, press the tofu between paper towels to get rid of the excess water, then cut into cubes.

Heat a large frying pan (or even better, a wok!) over a medium-high heat and add the sesame oil. The pan should be quite hot, but not overly spitting. Add the tofu and half the sauce. Fry until the tofu is golden, around 5–7 minutes. Remove the tofu from the pan and set aside.

Reduce the heat to medium and add the asparagus, carrot slices and spring onions to the pan with the rest of the sauce. Fry gently for 5 minutes. Add the kale and fry for 2 more minutes, then throw the tofu back in to warm it up.

Once you are sure all of the veggies are soft and cooked, serve on top of your drained, cooked quinoa.

Grilled Portobello Mushrooms with Roasted Sweetcorn Relish

1 garlic clove, minced
2 tablespoons olive oil
1 teaspoon dried oregano
4 large portobello mushrooms, stems removed
sea salt and freshly ground black pepper

For the Sweetcorn Relish
120g (¾ cup) sweetcorn (corn)
1 Romano (sweet) pepper, whole
2 tablespoons olive oil
2 tomatoes, roughly chopped
large handful of coriander (cilantro), roughly chopped
2 pinches of sea salt
2 pinches of freshly ground black pepper

Serves 4

I mentioned earlier that I've become obsessed with mushrooms because more and more studies are coming out about how amazing they are for our health. When I taste-tested this recipe I was so pleased with it that I made another batch for my husband. The relish is just so delicious, and if you have any left over, get some corn chips to dip in or a yummy piece of bread. Don't let it go to waste!

Preheat the grill (broiler) to medium-high. In a small bowl, whisk together the garlic, olive oil, oregano and salt and pepper until smooth, then coat the mushrooms in the mixture. Set aside.

Brush the sweetcorn and the Romano pepper with the olive oil and grill for 10 minutes, turning the pepper at least once. Remove and grill the mushrooms for 6 minutes, turning them over halfway through.

Roughly chop the grilled pepper and add to a bowl with the corn, tomatoes, coriander, salt and pepper, then mix well.

Take the portobello mushrooms out from under the grill and serve under a heap of the relish.

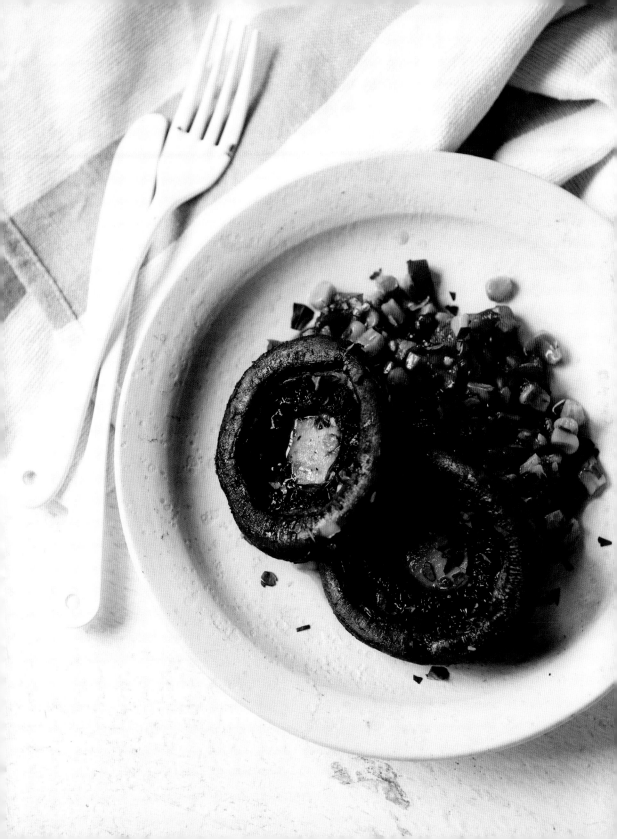

Walnut and Black Bean Wraps

1 x 400g tin (1⅔ cups) black beans, drained and rinsed
100g (heaping ⅔ cup) walnut halves
100g (scant 1 cup) sun-dried tomatoes
½ teaspoon ground cumin
½ teaspoon paprika
¼ teaspoon cayenne pepper, optional

To Serve
2 wholemeal (whole-wheat) tortillas
½ head romaine lettuce, shredded
½ avocado, peeled and sliced
juice of 1 lime
sea salt and freshly ground black pepper

Serves 2

This is the meatless burrito lunch that I've been making for a few years now, and it's a big hit with my kids, too (minus the cayenne pepper). Feel free to add additional toppings such as cheese or sour cream to make it a bit heartier, but these wraps are simply wonderful for a very quick lunch.

Blitz the black beans, walnuts, sun-dried tomatoes and spices in a food processor until the walnuts look like large crumbs.

Simply line the tortillas with the walnut and black bean taco 'meat', shredded lettuce and avocado. Squeeze the lime juice over each one and sprinkle with a little salt and pepper!

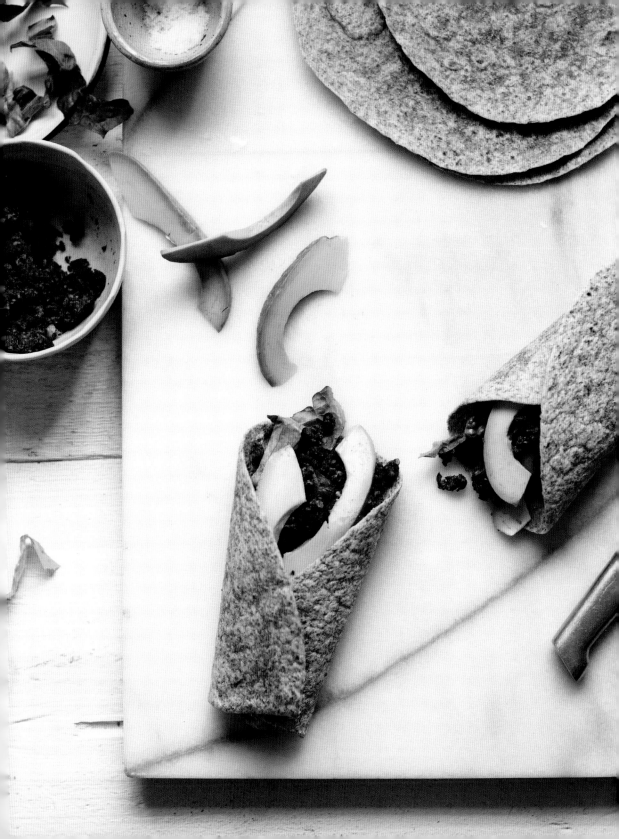

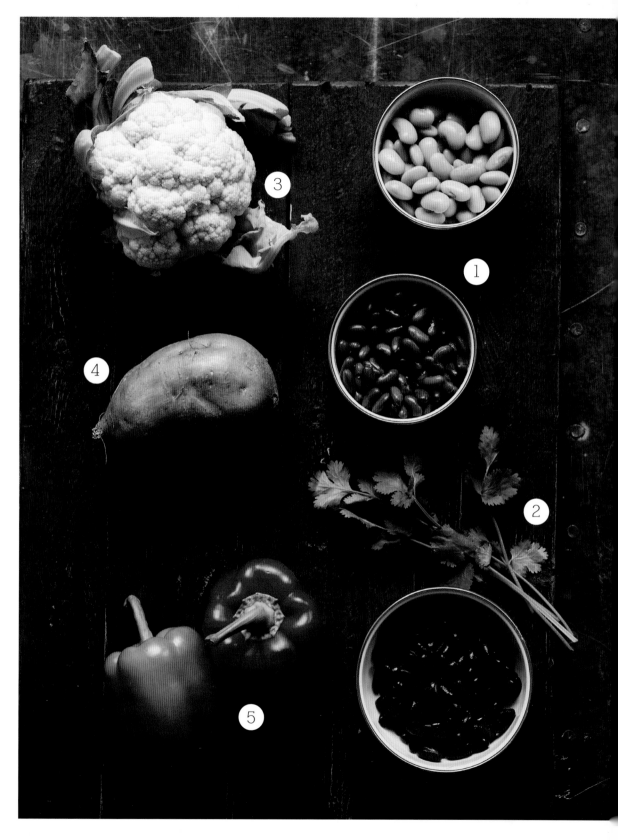

super SUPPERS

Pretty much every night for me needs to a superfast supper. Arriving home from a full day and having to feed four kids and still do loads of other things, such as helping them with their school work, getting them packed up for the next day, sports practice, piano, guitar... you see where I'm going with this. And in this wonderful modern world we live in, pretty much everyone I know is super-busy too. Unfortunately, one of the easiest things to let go of when life is like this is our food. Why? Because it's easy to pick up something 'already made', stick it in the microwave and boom! There's our supper in two minutes. But, believe it or not, when we eat these processed and packaged foods, it actually depletes our energy. So we are much, much better off carving out just 20 minutes every night to make something that will keep us healthy, happy and energized. Here are my top 20 superfast super-suppers.

superfood superheroes

1. Legumes (Black beans, cannellini, kidney beans, butter [lima] beans etc.)
There is a wide range of essential vitamins and minerals to be enjoyed by eating a variety of legumes. They are frequently referred to as an economical source of nutrition due to their low cost and abundance of goodness. Legumes are generally high in protein and fibre, low in fat, low in calories and contain no cholesterol. Aim to include as many different types of legumes as possible in order to enjoy the full effects!

2. Coriander (cilantro)
The natural chemical compounds in coriander are useful in preventing disease and promoting optimum health. The leaves are crammed full of antioxidants as well as being rich in a large number of essential vitamins and minerals.

3. Cauliflower
Cauliflower is a cruciferous vegetable that can be prepared in a range of ways. To get the maximum nutritional benefit it is best not to overcook it. Cauliflower consumption has

been linked to the prevention of certain cancers and is also often utilized for the detox support it provides to the body.

4. Sweet potatoes
Sweet potatoes have a much more interesting taste than regular potatoes, and many more health benefits! They are a particularly good source of vitamin A, which is linked to strong vision. Sweet potatoes contain a wealth of vitamins B6, C and D, all of which are essential to optimum function of the body in general. These amazing potatoes contain iron, potassium and magnesium, and will release natural sugars into the bloodstream slowly, helping to keep energy levels consistent.

5. (Bell) peppers
Peppers contain over 30 different compounds from the carotenoid family. These are plant pigments with important antioxidant properties. Bell peppers can help to balance blood sugar levels and contain quite an impressive amount of vitamins and minerals, while being low in fat.

Spicy Butter Bean Dhal

500ml (2 cups) vegetable stock
100g (½ cup + 1 tablespoon)
  uncooked split red lentils
1 onion, chopped
2 garlic cloves, crushed
1 teaspoon ground turmeric
1 teaspoon paprika
1 teaspoon ground cumin
½ teaspoon cayenne pepper
1 x 400g tin (1⅓ cups) butter
  (lima) beans, drained and
  rinsed
2 large handfuls of fresh
  spinach
wholemeal (whole-wheat)
  naan breads, to serve

Serves 4

Honestly, this one is SO easy that there is NO excuse not to make it. It's simply a case of chopping up some veg and popping it into a pot. And listen, if you don't have butter (lima) beans in your pantry, just swap them out for what you do have – chickpeas (garbanzo beans), white (haricot) beans and kidney beans all work just as well and taste great.

Place all the ingredients except the butter beans and spinach in a saucepan over a medium-high heat and bring to the boil. Add the butter beans, reduce the heat and simmer for 15 minutes.

Add the spinach and simmer for an additional 5 minutes, until the lentils are soft.

Serve with some yummy wholemeal naan breads and enjoy this super pot of healthy wholesomeness!

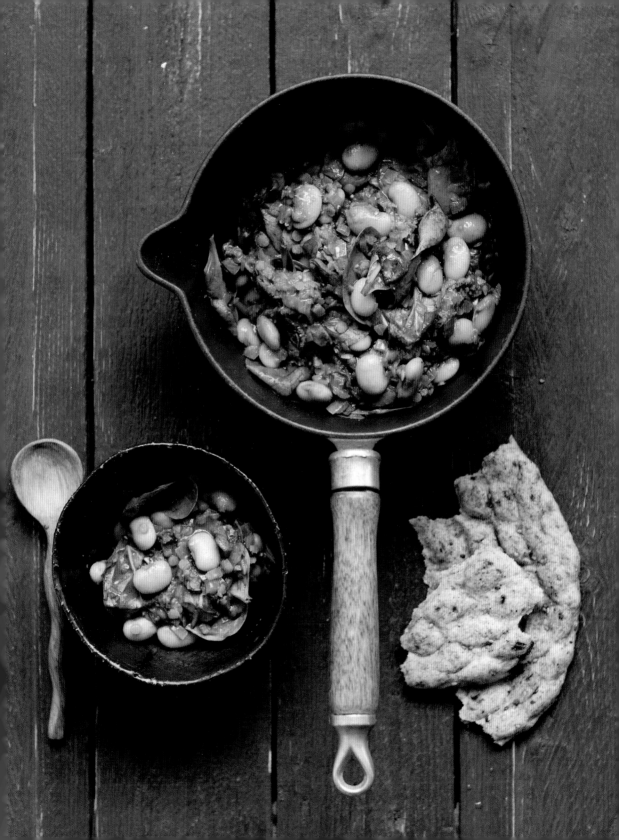

3-Bean Spicy Chilli

1 tablespoon coconut oil
1 onion, diced
3 garlic cloves, crushed
3 carrots, chopped
2 celery sticks, chopped
1 x 400g tin (1⅔ cups) white
  (haricot) beans, drained and
  rinsed
1 x 400g tin (1⅔ cups) black
  beans, drained and rinsed
1 x 400g tin (1⅔ cups) kidney
  beans, drained and rinsed
2 x 400g tins (3½ cups) chopped
  tomatoes
1 teaspoon chilli (chili) powder
½ teaspoon cayenne pepper
2 teaspoons ground cumin
small handful of basil,
  chopped
small handful of coriander
  (cilantro), roughly chopped
1 avocado, peeled, stoned and
  sliced
1 lime, quartered

Serves 4

Being American, chilli is a big deal for me. And growing up in the cold Chicago winters… well, chilli was an even bigger deal! Of course, chilli recipes ideally have meat in them, which of course is fine, but I've found that using different kinds of beans (there are three types in this recipe) makes a great and hearty substitute for the meat. So, on those cold, rainy days, let this heartwarming chilli be your failsafe, super-easy supper. Oh, and P.S., chilli freezes really well, so feel free to double this recipe so that you'll always have a batch on hand in a downpour.

In a large saucepan, melt the coconut oil over a medium-high heat, add the onion, garlic, carrot and celery and cook for 5 minutes.

Lower the heat to medium, add all the beans, chopped tomatoes and the spices and cook for 10 minutes. Lastly, stir in the basil until soft. This should only take a minute.

Spoon into bowls, garnish with the chopped coriander and top with the sliced avocado. Serve with lime wedges. It's SOOOO good!

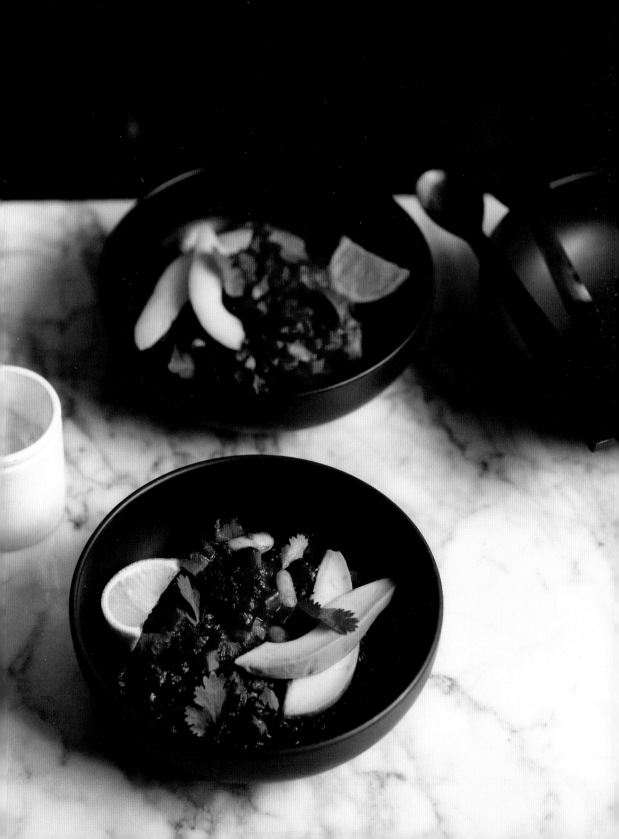

Kale Mac and Cheese

250g (2 cups) dried macaroni
(even better if it's gluten free
and/or wholegrain!)
1 tablespoon coconut oil
1 small onion, finely diced
2 garlic cloves, crushed
140g (heaping 1 cup) cashews,
soaked overnight, then
drained
350ml (1½ cups) almond
or coconut milk
1 tablespoon arrowroot
powder
25g (3 tablespoons) nutritional
yeast
½ teaspoon sweet paprika
½ teaspoon ground cumin
juice of ½ lemon
large handful of kale,
shredded

Serves 6

When I was growing up in the middle of America, I loved and lived on mac and cheese. I mean, let's be honest, it is just SO good! However, most mac and cheese isn't exactly going to give you what you need nutritionally and it depletes the energy supply. So, for my kids' sake, I had to find a mac and cheese that tasted as good (if not better) AND filled them with all things good. This recipe takes 20 minutes, but you do need to do a little planning and place the cashews in a bowl of water the night before. Then you're ready to go when you come home the next evening.

Cook the macaroni according to the packet instructions.

Meanwhile, heat a medium-sized saucepan over a medium heat, add the coconut oil and sauté the onion and garlic for 5 minutes or until soft.

Put the onion and garlic, soaked cashew nuts and the rest of the ingredients, except the kale, into a blender and blitz on high until thoroughly blended. Pour the cashew 'cheese' back into the saucepan with the shredded kale and cook on a low heat, stirring frequently, until warm and the kale is wilted – about 2–3 minutes.

Add the drained, cooked macaroni to the pan, stir well and serve immediately.

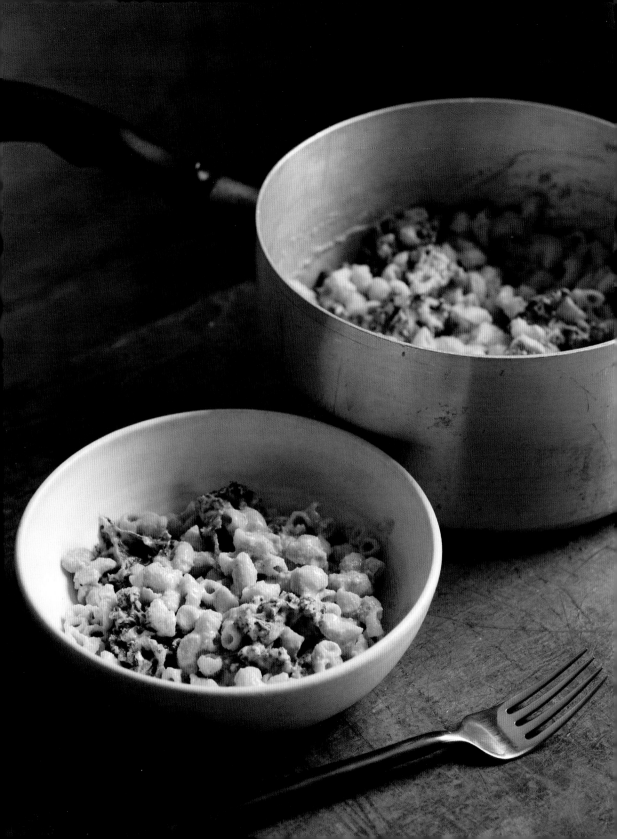

Portobello Mushroom Burger with Red Pepper Sauce

4 good-sized portobello
  mushrooms, stems removed
coconut oil, for brushing
1 large onion, thinly sliced
2 teaspoons coconut palm
  sugar
large handful of rocket
  (arugula)
4 gherkins, sliced in half
4 buns of your choice (I love
  wholemeal [whole-wheat]
  or gluten-free buns – maybe
  even toast the bun, too!)

For the Red Pepper Sauce
2 red (bell) peppers, seeds
  removed and sliced
coconut oil, for brushing
1 garlic clove, crushed
2 tablespoons olive oil
1 tablespoon apple cider
  vinegar
juice of 1 lemon
small handful of flaked
  (slivered) almonds
¼ teaspoon chilli flakes
  (red pepper flakes)
⅛ teaspoon chilli (chili) powder

Serves 4

I love a good veggie burger. When you find a recipe or a restaurant that has a good one, they are, to me, just as good as the traditional beef burger. But, to be honest, what makes burgers SO incredibly delicious is what you load them up with. So, this burger is simple, fast, delicious and the sauce is to die for!

Preheat the oven to 220°C/425°F/gas 7, using the fan if you have one. Brush the red pepper slices for the sauce with coconut oil and roast on a baking sheet for 10 minutes. Remove from the oven and allow to cool for a few minutes.

Meanwhile, brush the mushrooms with coconut oil and fry in a large frying pan over a medium-high heat for 5 minutes or until browned and soft. Remove with a slotted spoon and set aside. Add the thinly sliced onion to the same pan and cook for 5 minutes until soft. Add the coconut palm sugar and stir until dissolved and the onion caramelizes. Remove from the heat.

Once the red peppers have cooled, add them to a food processor or blender along with the rest of the ingredients for the red pepper sauce and blend until smooth.

Now, lay your lovely roasted mushrooms on the buns and slather on the delicious red pepper sauce (for me, the more the sauce the better). Top with equal amounts of the caramelized onion, gherkin halves and rocket.

It's just TOO yummy!

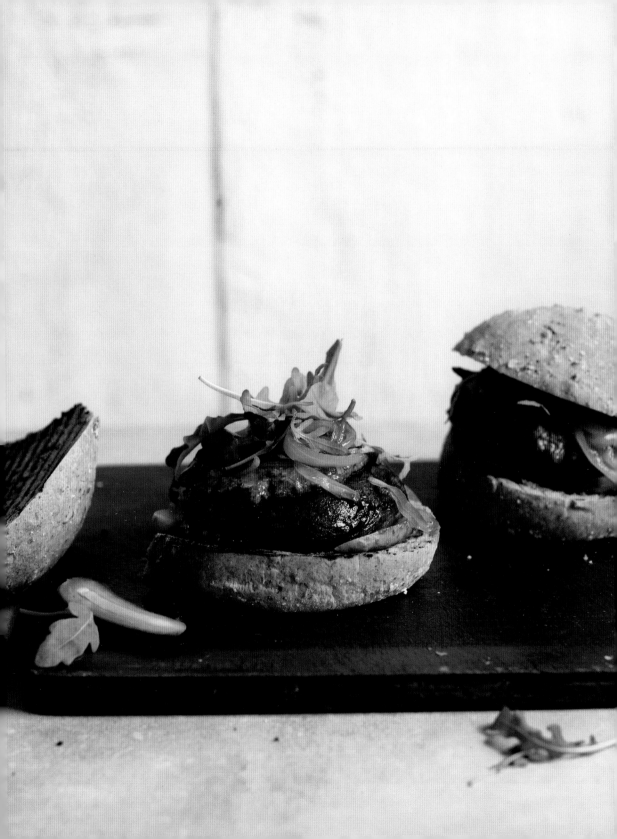

'Cheesey' Polenta and Black-eyed Beans Stir Fry

160g (1 cup) 'instant' or 'quick-cook' polenta
2 tablespoons coconut oil
1 large onion, sliced
2 garlic cloves, crushed
2 large carrots, shredded
150g (5½oz) Tenderstem broccoli (broccolini)
250g (1⅔ cups) cherry tomatoes, halved
1 x 400g tin (1¾ cups) black-eyed beans (peas), drained and rinsed
tamari or soy sauce, for drizzling

For the 'Cheese'
4 tablespoons nutritional yeast
2 tablespoons tamari or soy sauce
1 tablespoon tahini
1 tablespoon apple cider vinegar
juice of 1 lemon

Serves 4

I love polenta, but most people I've spoken with find it tasteless and I have to agree. But the thing about polenta is that it really is nutritionally very, very good for us. However, it rarely finds itself on our plates at home. So, this recipe came from some deep thinking as to how to get this good-for-you (and inexpensive) grain into our diets more.

In a small bowl, whisk together the 'cheese' ingredients until smooth.

Cook the polenta according to the packet instructions. (As long as you have the instant/quick-cook polenta, this will just take a few minutes.)

In a large frying pan or wok, heat the coconut oil over a medium-high heat. Add the onion, garlic and carrots and cook for 5 minutes until soft, stirring occasionally. Reduce the heat to medium and add the broccoli, tomatoes and black-eyed beans with a drizzle of tamari or soy sauce to help the veg cook. Continue to cook for about 8 minutes, stirring occasionally.

Spoon the polenta onto plates, drizzle with the 'cheese' sauce, top with the stir fry and dig in!

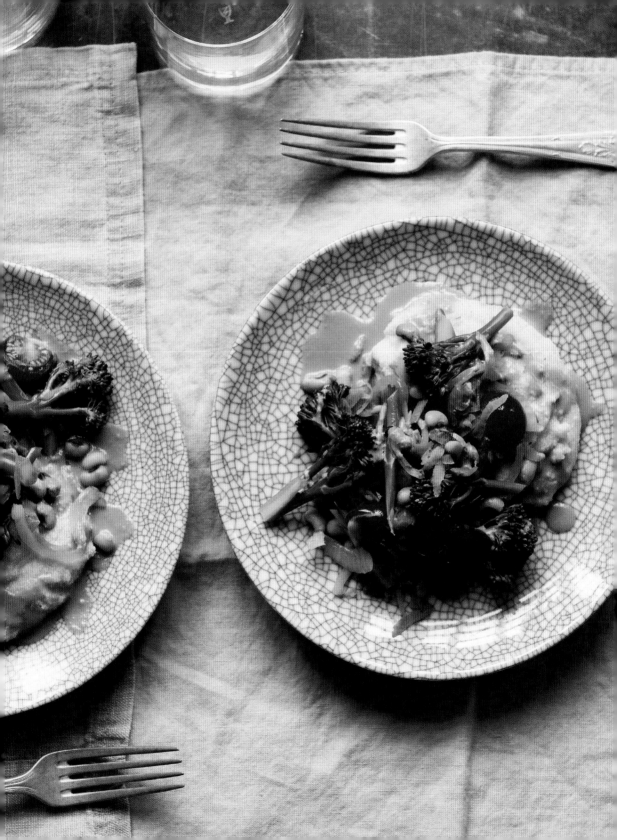

Cauliflower Rice and Almond Tofu with Greens

350g (12oz) firm tofu
2 tablespoons sesame oil
2 garlic cloves, crushed
60ml (¼ cup) tamari or soy
  sauce
3 tablespoons honey
3 tablespoons almond butter
1 large cauliflower head
120g (3–4 small bunches) baby
  pak choi (bok choy)
2 tablespoons coconut oil
2 spring onions (scallions),
  chopped

Serves 4

A super-fast alternative to cooking rice is cauliflower. I know, it might not sound very appealing at first, but try this recipe and you might just be converted. And I always think it's more fun to go for something different every once in a while. Of course, feel free to use brown rice instead... but I have a feeling that once you have tried this new kind of rice, you might never look back!

Begin by placing the tofu between a few paper towels and pressing with your hands to release the water.

Preheat the oven to 200°C/400°F/gas 6 and line a baking sheet with parchment paper.

In a small bowl, combine the sesame oil, crushed garlic, tamari or soy sauce, honey and almond butter. Put to one side.

Cut the cauliflower into chunks and place it in a food processor. Pulse until it resembles rice. Heat a large frying pan over a medium heat and add the cauliflower rice, baby pak choi and the coconut oil. Stir to combine, cover and cook for 5–8 minutes until the cauliflower and pak choi are tender.

Place the tofu on the prepared baking sheet in a single layer and coat with the almond butter mixture. Bake for 10 minutes. Once cooked, add the tofu to the cauliflower rice and pak choi. Serve on warm plates and sprinkle with the spring onions.

Fried Quinoa

270g (1½ cups) uncooked
   quinoa, well rinsed
400ml (1¾ cups) vegetable
   stock
2 tablespoons coconut oil
2 spring onions (scallions),
   thinly sliced
1 tablespoon minced fresh
   ginger
3 garlic cloves, crushed
1 small onion, finely diced
small broccoli head, cut into
   florets
1 sweet potato, peeled and
   finely chopped
1 red (bell) pepper, seeds
   removed and finely chopped
3 tablespoons tamari
1 tablespoon sesame oil
small handful of coriander
   (cilantro), chopped
2 large handfuls of kale,
   shredded
2 tablespoons sesame seeds
1 lime, quartered

Serves 4

Honestly, my kids love fried rice and – actually – so do I. However, I think most of us know that the MSG (monosodium glutamate) that is found in most fried rice isn't so good for us! So, no, this recipe has no MSG, and I could easily have made it with brown rice, but there's something about the high amounts of protein in quinoa that, for me, makes it feel more like a main meal.

In a large saucepan over a high heat, combine the quinoa and veggie stock and bring to the boil. Reduce the heat, cover and simmer for 15 minutes until cooked.

Meanwhile, add the coconut oil, spring onions, ginger, garlic and onion to a large frying pan over a high heat, stirring for 2–3 minutes. Add the broccoli, sweet potato and red pepper and continue to cook for 3 minutes.

Once the quinoa is cooked, add it to the vegetable mixture along with the tamari and sesame oil and cook for a further 5 minutes. Stir in the coriander and kale and cook for another minute, until the kale has wilted.

Sprinkle with the sesame seeds and serve with the lime wedges on the side.

Coconut Quinoa Curry

170g (scant 1 cup) uncooked
quinoa, well rinsed
1 x 400ml tin (1¾ cups) coconut
milk
juice of 1 lime

For the Sauce
1 tablespoon coconut oil
1 onion, diced
2 garlic cloves, chopped
2.5-cm (1-inch) piece fresh
ginger, peeled and finely
chopped
1 x 400ml tin (1¾ cups) coconut
milk
1 tablespoon curry powder
200ml (¾ cup + 1½ tablespoons)
vegetable stock
1 small broccoli head,
cut into florets
1 red (bell) pepper, seeds
removed and sliced
1 orange (bell) pepper, seeds
removed and sliced
75g (⅔ cup) frozen peas

Serves 2

Yup, curry, but with a different grain – not your typical rice. Quinoa is again a great grain to cook on those days you need a fast, easy and healthy meal. I'm loving the addition of the ginger here as well and there's a lot of it, too! So, if you are feeing a bit run down, this should be your supper choice because ginger does the body worlds of good.

In a medium saucepan over a high heat, add the quinoa, coconut milk and lime juice. Bring to the boil, reduce the heat to a simmer, cover and cook for 15 minutes until all the liquid has been absorbed.

Meanwhile, heat a medium saucepan over a medium heat and melt the coconut oil. Add in the onion, garlic and ginger. Stir for a few minutes and then add the coconut milk, curry powder and vegetable stock. Stir for 1 minute.

Add the broccoli, peppers and peas and cook for 10 minutes, stirring occasionally. After this time the quinoa should be cooked, so you can now drain any excess liquid if necessary. Serve with the coconut curry.

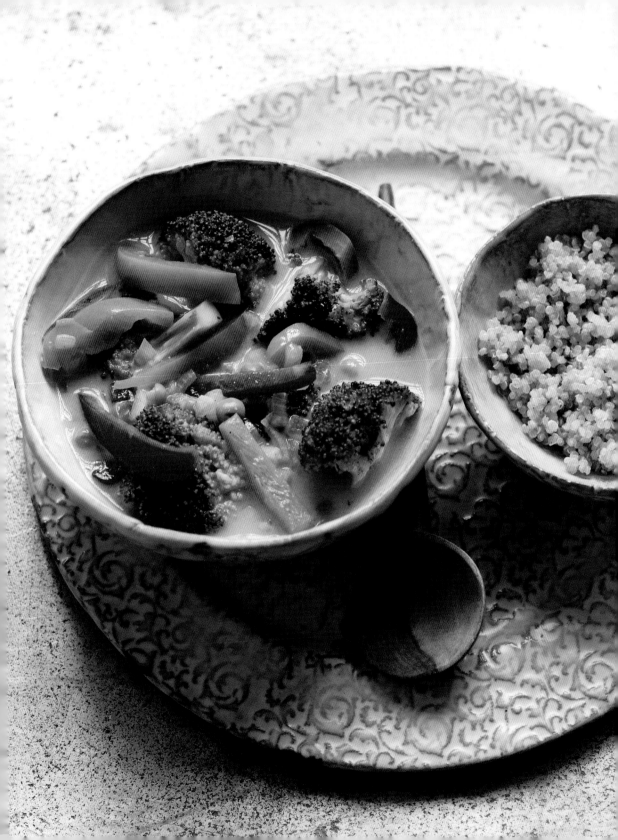

Green Risotto

350g (12oz) asparagus spears
80g (⅔ cup) petits pois (French peas)
4 tablespoons coconut oil
375g (2¼ cups) uncooked buckwheat
1 small onion, roughly diced
1 litre (4¼ cups) vegetable stock
50ml (3½ tablespoons) apple cider vinegar
large handful of basil
sea salt and freshly ground black pepper

Serves 4

Those that know me know that I love greens. I seriously try to get at least one green veg into my diet every single day, no matter what. Greens are great for the liver, which is wonderful, but I love them because they are also incredibly energizing. And I need and want as much energy as I can get. So here's a quick and easy risotto that's a bit different from typical recipes because it's all about the greens.

Fill a medium saucepan with water and bring to the boil. Cut the ends off the asparagus and discard, then slice into 3-cm (1¼-inch) chunks. Place in the boiling water with the petits pois for 3 minutes. Drain and rinse.

Meanwhile, add the coconut oil, buckwheat, onion, veg stock and apple cider vinegar to a large frying pan over a medium-high heat. Stir until the coconut oil has melted and then cook at a slight boil for 15 minutes.

While the buckwheat is cooking, add half the petits pois and asparagus along with the basil and 100ml (⅓ cup) water to a food processor or blender and blend until smooth. Mix the purée into the buckwheat risotto, season with salt and pepper, garnish with the remaining petits pois and asparagus pieces and serve!

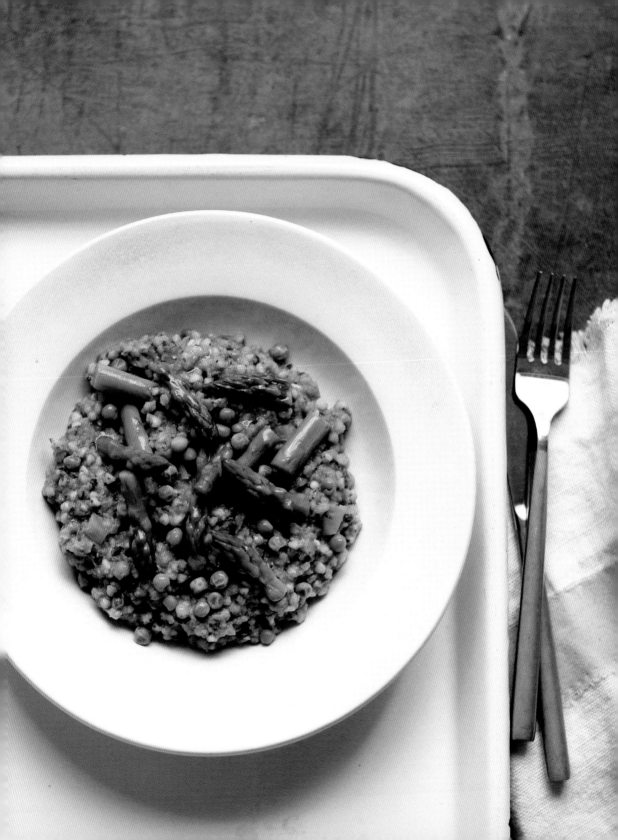

Brown Rice Bowl

200g (1 heaping cup) brown
  rice
720ml (1½ pints) vegetable
  stock
2 large handfuls pitted black
  or kalamata olives, roughly
  chopped
2 tablespoons olive oil
90g (⅔ cup) walnut halves
  (toasted, if preferred)
small handful of dill
½ teaspoon chilli flakes
  (red pepper flakes)
juice of 1 lemon
2 tablespoons honey
50g (heaping ⅓ cup) dried
  cranberries
4 spring onions (scallions),
  chopped
sea salt and freshly ground
  black pepper

Serves 4

I always think the 'B' in brown rice stands for vitamin B because, of all the grains, brown rice contains the most of this important vitamin. So on those days when you feel like you need a vitamin B injection, this is the bowl for you.

Bring the brown rice and stock to the boil in a saucepan over a medium-high heat. Boil until the rice is tender and cooked, about 15 minutes. Drain off any excess water, if necessary.

Meanwhile, place the olives in a bowl with the rest of the ingredients. Season, stir well and refrigerate until the rice is cooked.

Combine the rice and olive and walnut mixture, stir well and eat well, too!

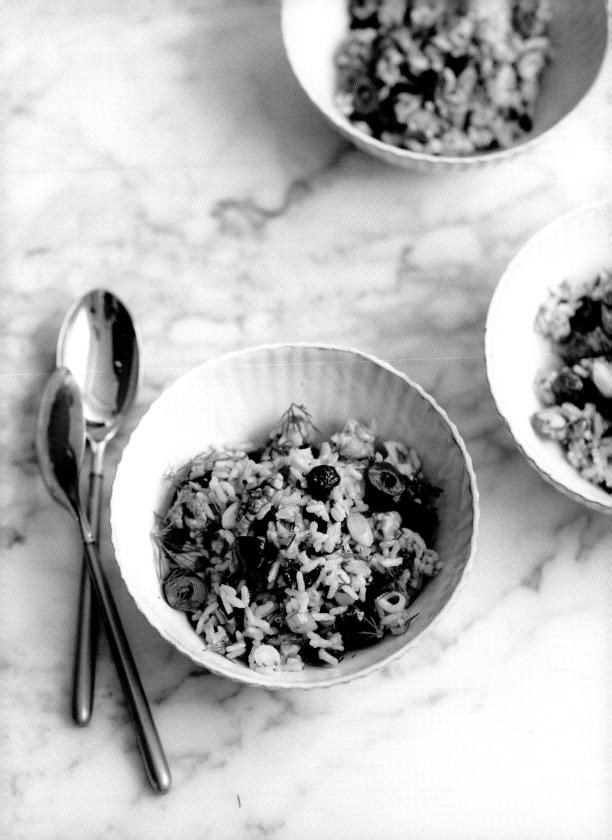

Ginger Tahini and Mint Pasta

500g (18oz) of your favourite
dried pasta
2 garlic cloves, crushed
2 tablespoons grated fresh
ginger
4 tablespoons tahini
2 tablespoons tamari or soy
sauce
2 tablespoons apple cider
vinegar
2 tablespoons honey
juice of 1 lime
large handful of mint, roughly
torn
sea salt and freshly ground
black pepper

Serves 4

Want something bigger, better and healthier than your easy pasta with tomato sauce? Well, this pasta sauce is simple, yet just out of this world! On those nights when all you can manage is boiling some water and pushing the button on the food processor, this is your go-to, healthy and yummy meal.

Cook the pasta according to the packet instructions.

Meanwhile, place all the other ingredients, reserving a few mint leaves, in a food processor or blender and whizz until smooth.

Stir the sauce into the drained cooked pasta and serve in bowls, garnished with the reserved mint.

Now, that's what I call easy!

Mexican Black Bean Burgers

2 tablespoons coconut oil
2 shallots, finely grated
2 garlic cloves, crushed
1 x 400g tin (1⅔ cups) black
  beans, drained and rinsed
2 green chillies (chile peppers),
  seeds removed and chopped
1 teaspoon ground cumin
½ teaspoon chilli (chili) powder
1 tablespoon olive oil
½ teaspoon cayenne pepper
large handful of coriander
  (cilantro), chopped
juice of 1 lime
2 tablespoons ground flaxseed
  (linseed)
sea salt and freshly ground
  black pepper

To Serve
toasted buns
sliced avocado
sliced red onion
salsa

Serves 2

I could probably eat a Mexican dish every single day. I love the spices, I love the beans, I love the avocado, I love the salsa – I just love Mexican food! This is my tribute to a veggie burger... but this one has that Mexican bite. It's super simple and super spicy! Feel free to add some corn tortilla chips and salsa to make it even more Mexican.

Heat a medium frying pan over a medium heat and melt 1 tablespoon of the coconut oil. Add the shallots and garlic and cook for 2 minutes, or until soft, then transfer to a mixing bowl along with the drained black beans, green chillies, cumin, chilli powder, olive oil, cayenne pepper, coriander, lime juice, flaxseed and seasoning. Using a fork, mash the ingredients together to combine. Add more oil or lime juice if it's too dry.

Divide the mixture into two and shape into patties. Using the same pan over a medium heat, melt the remaining coconut oil and cook the burgers for 4 minutes on each side, flipping very gently.

Serve on toasted buns and top with sliced avocado, sliced red onion and salsa.

Spicy Tofu Tacos

2 tablespoons coconut oil
1 large red onion, diced
2 garlic cloves, crushed
1 red (bell) pepper, seeds
  removed and finely sliced
1 yellow (bell) pepper, seeds
  removed and finely sliced
250g (9oz) firm tofu
1 x 400g tin (1⅔ cups) black
  beans, drained and rinsed
2 green chillies (chile peppers),
  seeds removed and roughly
  chopped
1 teaspoon chilli (chili) powder
1 teaspoon cayenne pepper
2 limes
large handful of coriander
  (cilantro), roughly chopped
2 spring onions (scallions),
  chopped
sea salt and freshly ground
  black pepper

To Serve
8 corn tortillas
coconut or soya yogurt,
  optional

Serves 4

For 'Meatless Mondays', this is one of my favourite dishes. You can make this as spicy as you want or you can just as easily leave out the spice altogether. You've got whole grains from the corn tortilla, protein from the tofu and a good amount of veggies, too.

In a large frying pan over a medium-high heat, melt the coconut oil, add the onion, garlic and red and yellow peppers and then cook for about 3 minutes, stirring occasionally.

Crumble the tofu into the pan and stir, scraping the bottom of the pan when needed. After 10 minutes, add the black beans, green chillies, chilli powder and cayenne. Stir well and continue to cook for 2 minutes. Season to taste.

Squeeze the lime juice into the pan, sprinkle with the coriander and spring onions and serve with the corn tortillas, topping with the yogurt, if using.

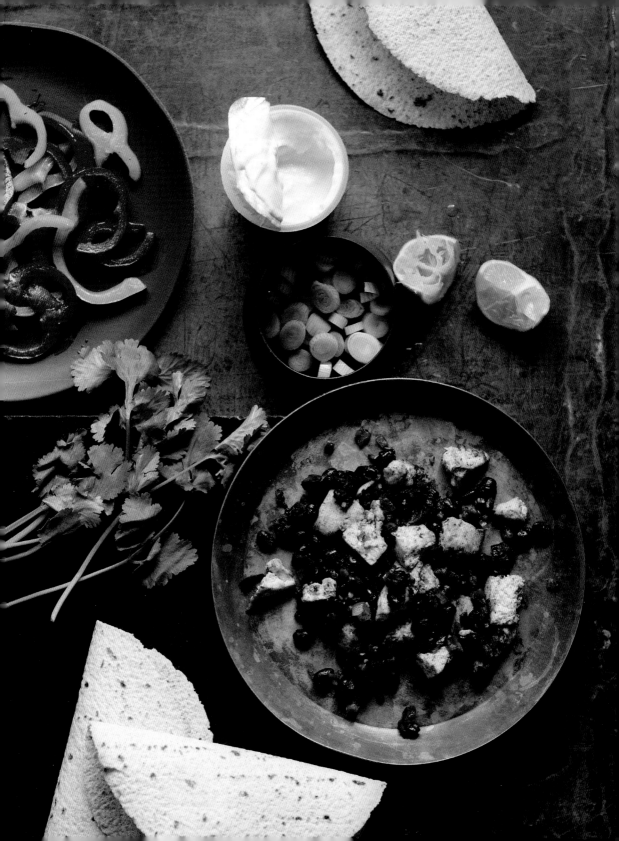

Julie's Sloppy Joes

1 tablespoon olive oil
1 large onion, finely diced
1 garlic clove, crushed
1 x 400g tin (14oz) lentils,
  drained and rinsed
1 x 400g tin (1¾ cups) chopped
  tomatoes
2 tablespoons tomato purée
  (paste)
1 tablespoon maple syrup or
  honey
1 teaspoon chilli (chili) powder
1 teaspoon sweet paprika
60ml (¼ cup) water or
  vegetable stock
sea salt and freshly ground
  black pepper
4 buns (preferably wholemeal/
  wheat or gluten free), to serve

Serves 4

Growing up in America, Sloppy Joes were a staple meal at home and even at restaurants. And my mum made the best! So, here is a veggie twist on an American classic that, frankly, I think is just as good as my mum's!

Heat the olive oil in a large saucepan over a medium-high heat. Cook the onion and garlic for 5 minutes until soft, then add the rest of the ingredients, season to taste and mix well. Bring to the boil and then reduce the heat and simmer for 10 minutes, or until the mixture thickens to your liking.

Serve in the buns and enjoy the sloppiness of the Sloppy Joe!

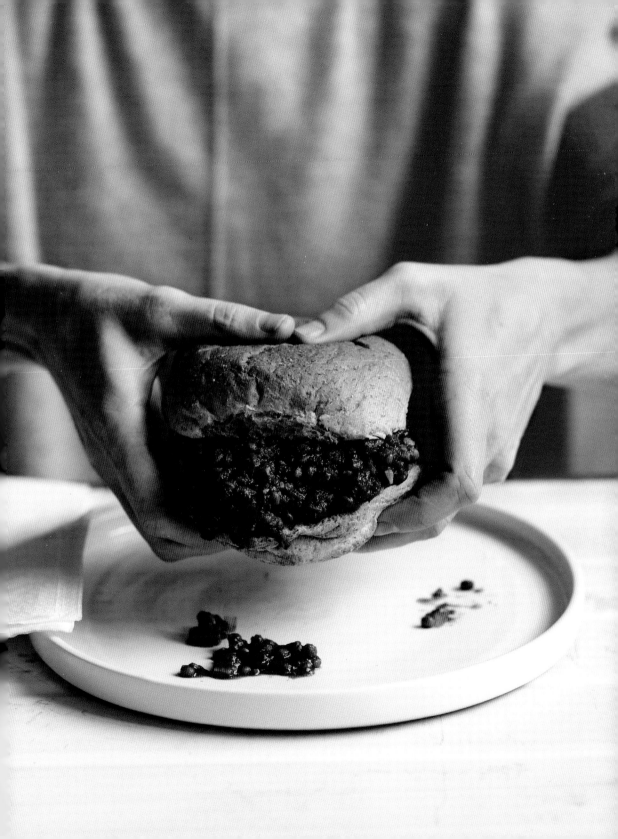

Perfect Pasta Primavera

250g (9oz) of your preferred dried pasta (I like quinoa and corn pastas, which are both gluten free)
2 tablespoons coconut or olive oil
1 onion, roughly chopped
2 garlic cloves, crushed
1 courgette (zucchini), roughly chopped
1 small aubergine (eggplant), roughly chopped
130g (1⅓ cups) pitted black and kalamata olives
1 x 400ml tin (1¾ cups) chopped tomatoes
2 tablespoons tomato purée (paste)
1 teaspoon ground cumin
1 teaspoon sweet paprika
½ teaspoon cayenne pepper
½ teaspoon chilli (chili) powder
1 teaspoon chilli flakes (red pepper flakes)
juice of 1 lemon
handful of basil, chopped
sea salt and freshly ground black pepper

Serves 4

Yes, you can make this perfect pasta sauce in just under 20 minutes and it's filled with all things good, too. So rather than grabbing that jar of sauce that's most likely filled with a lot of sugar and salt, take 20 minutes out and fill your body and mind with something that's, in my view, rather perfect!

Cook the pasta according to the packet instructions.

Meanwhile, heat the oil in a large saucepan over a medium-high heat and sauté the onion and garlic for 3 minutes. Add the courgette, aubergine and olives and cook for another minute. Mix in the tinned tomatoes, tomato purée, cumin, sweet paprika, cayenne pepper, chilli powder, chilli flakes and lemon juice and season with salt and pepper. Reduce the heat to medium, cover the pan and cook for an additional 10–12 minutes, stirring every few minutes, until the veggies are tender.

Remove from heat and mix the sauce into the drained cooked pasta. Garnish with the chopped basil.

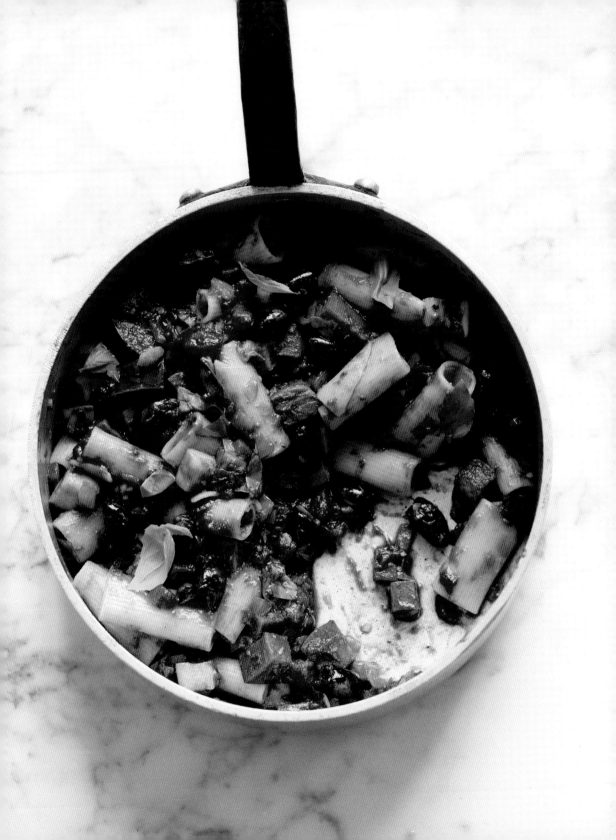

Courgetti Spaghetti with White Beans and Chia Pesto

125g (4½oz) dried spaghetti
  (gluten free or wholegrain)
1 x 400g tin (1⅔ cups) white
  (haricot) beans, drained
  and rinsed
1 onion, finely chopped
2 garlic cloves, crushed
4 large handfuls of fresh
  spinach
2 tablespoons olive oil
juice of 1 lemon
2 large courgettes (zucchini),
  spiralized
large handful of basil,
  leaves torn
sea salt and freshly ground
  black pepper

For the Chia Pesto
35g (¼ cup) pine nuts
35g (¼ cup) walnut halves
2 garlic cloves, crushed
100g (3½oz) basil, stems
  removed
4 tablespoons olive oil
2 tablespoons chia seeds
2 tablespoons nutritional yeast
2 tablespoons apple cider
  vinegar
juice of 1 lemon

spiralizer

Serves 4

As you can see from the recipes in this book, I love food, particularly healthy and hearty food. And so for me, when I want a main meal using spiralized courgettes (zucchini), a heartier meal is actually combining courgette noodles with spaghetti! You're getting some great vitamins and minerals from the veg, beans and chia in this supper, along with the energy that comes form the carbs in the pasta. In my book, that's pretty perfect.

Cook the pasta according to the packet instructions.

Meanwhile, add the beans, onion, garlic, spinach, olive oil and lemon juice to a large saucepan over a medium heat. Cook until the spinach wilts, about 5 minutes.

Add the drained cooked pasta and the spiralized courgette to the bean mixture and keep on low heat. Season to taste.

Blend all the pesto ingredients in a food processor or blender until smooth, then add to the pan and mix to coat the pasta mixture.

Scatter the torn basil leaves over the top and serve.

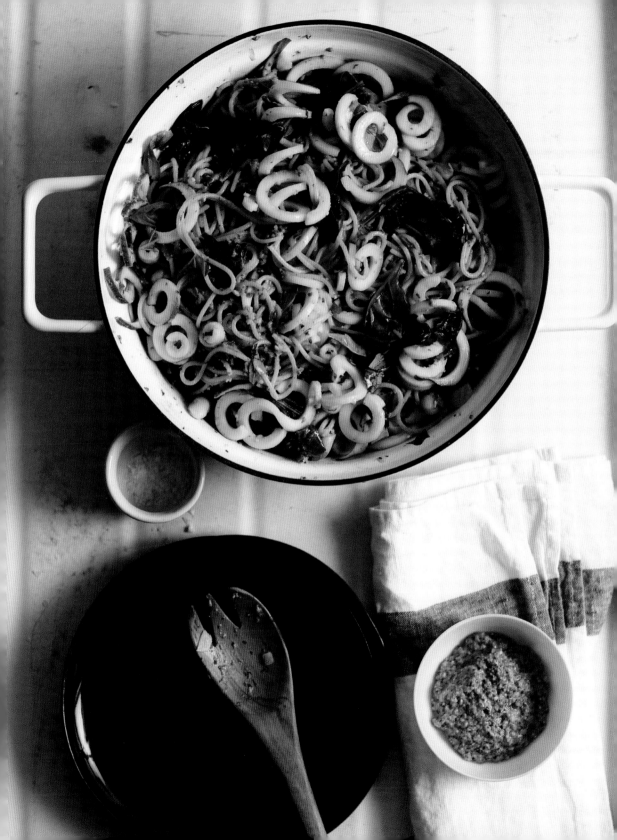

Sweet Potato and Black Bean Burritos

4 small sweet potatoes, peeled and roughly chopped
1 tablespoon coconut oil
1 onion, chopped
2 garlic cloves, crushed
1 red (bell) pepper, seeds removed and chopped
1 x 400g tin (1⅔ cups) black beans, drained and rinsed
juice of 1 lime
1 teaspoon chilli (chili) powder
1 teaspoon ground cumin
4 wholemeal (whole-wheat) tortillas

For the Avocado Cream
1 avocado, peeled and stoned
1 garlic clove, crushed
large handful of coriander (cilantro)
120ml (½ cup) coconut or soya yogurt
2 tablespoons lime juice
1 tablespoon honey
sea salt and freshly ground black pepper

Serves 4

I know what you're thinking… how can cooking sweet potatoes take 20 minutes or less? Well, it can! You just need to boil them like you would white potatoes. The sweet potato combined with the black beans almost makes this seem rather meaty. It's super filling, super healthy and the sauce is super amazing!

Place the sweet potatoes in a medium saucepan. Fill with enough water to cover and bring to the boil over a medium-high heat. Boil for 7 minutes, at which point they should be tender.

Meanwhile, heat the coconut oil in a large frying pan over a medium-high heat. Add the onion and garlic and sauté for 5 minutes. Drain the sweet potatoes and add them to the pan along with the red pepper, black beans, lime juice and spices. Cook over a medium-high heat for another 5 minutes. Take the pan off the heat and mash the sweet potatoes and beans, but keep them 'chunky'. Layer the tortillas with the sweet potato and black bean mixture.

Add all the ingredients for the avocado cream to a food processor or blender and blitz until smooth.

Spread the avocado cream on top of the sweet potato mixture and fold the tortillas to make burritos.

Miso Mushroom Soba Noodles

250g (9oz) uncooked soba
   noodles
2 tablespoons coconut oil
1 onion, finely sliced into half
   moons
2 garlic cloves, crushed
125g (4½oz) oyster mushrooms
125g (4½oz) shiitake
   mushrooms
125g baby pak choi (bok choy)
2 tablespoons miso paste
2 tablespoons tamari or soy
   sauce
2 teaspoons chilli flakes
   (red pepper flakes)
2 spring onions (scallions),
   chopped
2 tablespoons black sesame
   seeds
sea salt and freshly ground
   black pepper

Serves 4

I truly believe it when I read that mushrooms have medicinal qualities. One of their superhero properties is vitamin D, and it's the only vegetarian food source of this vital vitamin. Considering that vitamin D deficiency is thought to be quite widespread in the western world, this is a great way to get it through your food.

Firstly, prepare the soba noodles according to the packet instructions.

Meanwhile, melt the coconut oil in a medium frying pan over a medium-high heat and cook the onion and garlic for 5 minutes until soft. While they are softening, clean and slice the mushrooms, then add them to the pan with a pinch of salt and pepper and continue to fry for 5 minutes.

While the mushrooms are cooking, slice the pak choi, then add it to the pan and fry for another 5 minutes. Add the miso, tamari or soy sauce and chilli flakes and fry for 1 more minute. Finally, add the drained cooked soba noodles and sprinkle the spring onions and black sesame seeds over the top.

Divide between four bowls and serve!

Cannellini Bean Masala

2 tablespoons coconut oil
1 red onion, diced
1 yellow (bell) pepper, seeds
   removed and chopped
1 small cauliflower head,
   cut into florets
1 medium courgette (zucchini),
   cut into bite-sized chunks
1 tablespoon garam masala
1½ teaspoons ground cumin
1½ teaspoons ground turmeric
1 x 400g tin (1¾ cups) chopped
   tomatoes
1 x 400g tin (1⅓ cups) cannellini
   beans, drained and rinsed
1 x 400ml tin (1¾ cups) coconut
   milk
240ml (1 cup) vegetable stock
large handful of coriander
   (cilantro), chopped, optional
sea salt and freshly ground
   black pepper
pappadums or naan breads,
   to serve

Serves 4

This is a new twist on the masala. And there is the option to add brown rice, quinoa or even millet to this recipe – all these grains take 15–20 minutes to cook – although I found this recipe super filling all on its own. The coconut milk makes it thick and creamy and I just eat it with pappadums or naan bread to scoop out the last few mouthfuls. Super easy, super yummy!

Melt the coconut oil in a large saucepan over a medium-high heat. Add the red onion, yellow pepper, cauliflower and courgette and cook for 3 minutes. Add the spices, mix well and cook for another minute. Stir in the tomatoes and cannellini beans. Mix well, cover and cook for 5 minutes.

Stir in the coconut milk and veggie stock and reduce the heat to medium. Cook for 2 more minutes, top with the coriander, if using, and serve in bowls with pappadums or warm naan breads on the side.

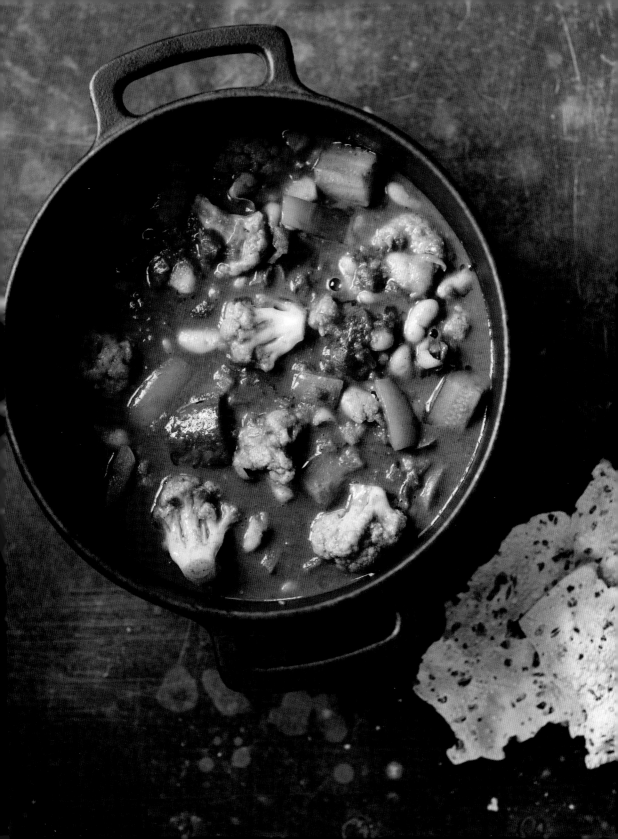

Artichoke, Mushroom and Kidney Bean Millet with a Lemon Tahini Dressing

200g (1 cup) uncooked millet
2 tablespoons coconut oil
1 red onion, diced
1 garlic clove, thinly sliced
1 large celery stick, chopped
300g (4½ cups) button
  mushrooms, sliced
280g (10oz) tinned artichoke
  hearts, drained, rinsed and
  halved
1 x 400g tin (1⅔ cups) kidney
  beans, drained and rinsed
large handful of pumpkin
  seeds
handful of parsley, chopped
sea salt and freshly ground
  black pepper
toasted rye bread, to serve,
  optional

For the dressing
2 garlic cloves, crushed
2 heaping tablespoons tahini
2 tablespoons nutritional yeast
2 tablespoons olive oil
1 tablespoon apple cider
  vinegar
juice of 1 lemon
small handful of parsley

Serves 4

This might be one of my favourite Super Supper recipes and that's partially due to the fact that I LOVE artichokes and mushrooms… equally. I wanted to find a fast recipe to incorporate both of them. Millet is a quick and nutritious grain to add to the dressing and, well, I'll let you be the judge but for me, it's a recipe to come back to time and time again.

Cook the millet according to the packet instructions, about 15 minutes. It's a quick grain to cook!

Meanwhile, melt the coconut oil in a large saucepan over a medium-high heat. Add the red onion and garlic and fry for 5 minutes. Add the celery, mushrooms, artichokes and beans and fry for a further 5 minutes, stirring occasionally. Place all the dressing ingredients in a food processor or blender and blitz until smooth.

In a large bowl, combine the millet with the mushroom and artichoke mixture and mix well. Season to taste. Drizzle over the dressing, stir it in well and sprinkle with the pumpkin seeds and parsley.

Serve with toasted rye bread, if you like, to make a more substantial supper dish. And there you have it – quick, easy and super delicious!

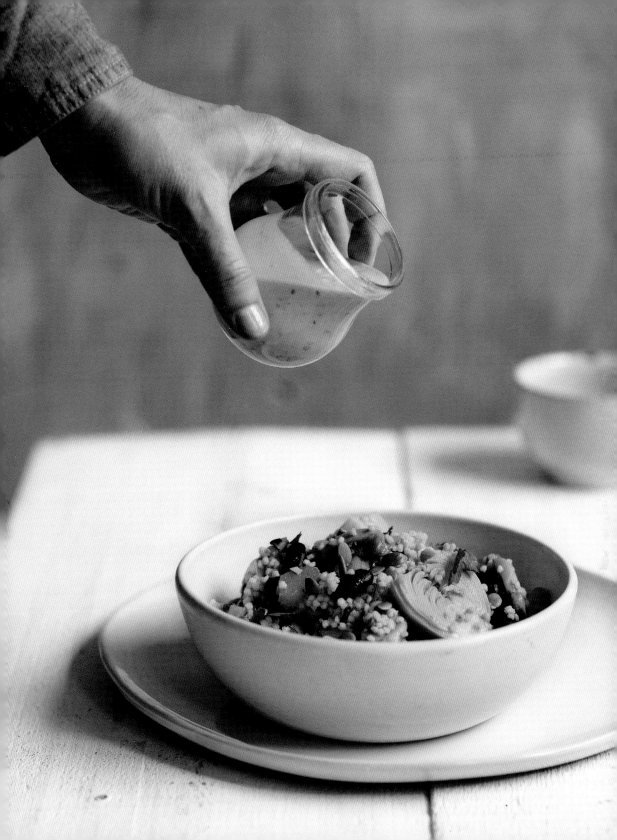

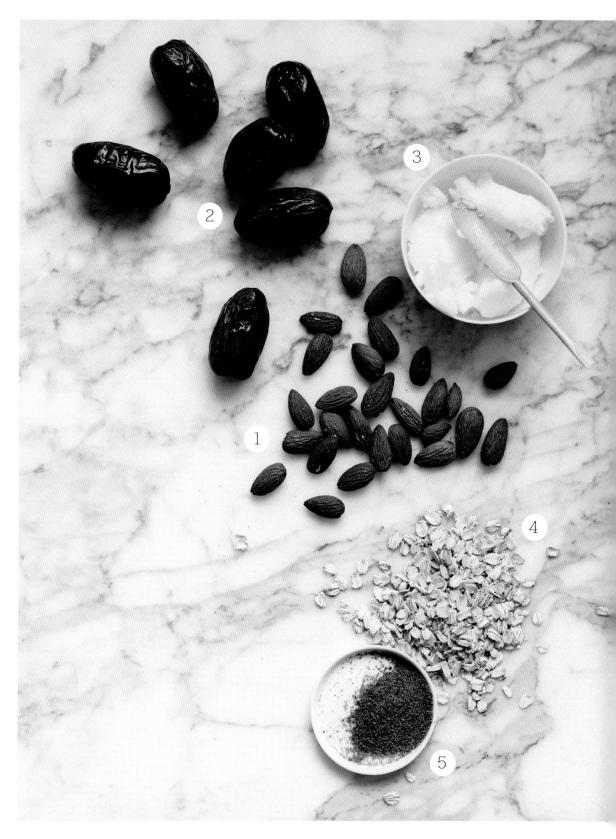

super SWEETS

When I was writing this chapter, my youngest asked me what my favourite recipe in this section is. I looked through all of the recipes with every intention of telling him that there was a clear winner, but my taste buds wouldn't let me! Because every time, I thought, 'Yes, this one!' I'd see the next recipe and remember how delicious that one was, too! So, I hope you thoroughly enjoy these Super Sweet recipes as much as I do.

superfood superheroes

1. Almonds
A handful of almonds will provide your body with an adequate amount of fibre, protein, vitamin E, manganese and magnesium. They also contain a generous amount of copper and phosphorous. Almonds are perfect to include in your diet as a snack between meals and can be used in main meals, salads and desserts!

2. Dates
Dates are the perfect natural snack food for anyone with a sweet tooth. They have quite a chewy consistency that makes them great for baking to bind foods together. Dates are crammed with vitamins and minerals, and are also easy to digest, which means that your body can make use of the goodness contained within!

3. Coconut oil
Coconut oil is one of the healthiest oils you can cook with and packed full of heart-healthy fats. It is linked with improved digestion as well as weight loss, especially in the abdominal region. As well as boosting the function of your metabolism, coconut oil can also improve your immune system and combat sugar cravings. Not only is it good for your insides, but it also does wonders for the skin and can help to keep wrinkles at bay for longer when used topically.

4. Oats
Oats are one of the best breakfast options you can choose when it comes to preserving the health of your body. They contain a unique group of antioxidants known as avenanthramides, which are thought to provide powerful protection for the heart. Oats are low in calories and fat while being high in fibre, protein and complex carbohydrates.

5. Coconut palm sugar
Coconut palm sugar is made from the sap of the coconut tree and is becoming increasingly popular as a natural sweetener. It is thought to be a better alternative to other sugars for people with diabetes as long as the product is 100% coconut palm sugar and not mixed with other products. There is also a range of trace vitamins and minerals in this sugar as well as small amounts of various phytonutrients.

Lentil Brownies

coconut oil, for greasing
2 x 400g tins (1¾lb) lentils,
  drained and rinsed
4 tablespoons almond butter
1 small banana
4 tablespoons raw cacao
  powder, plus extra for dusting
1 tablespoon honey
½ teaspoon bicarbonate of
  soda (baking soda)
12 Medjool dates (make sure
  you are using soft dates and
  Medjools are the softest!),
  pitted

20 x 20-cm (8 x 8-inch) baking
  tin

Makes 12

Okay, I know this might sound a bit weird and you might be asking, 'Is she serious?' But yes, I am serious! I urge you to try this because I promise you, these brownies are seriously good and gooey! They do not disappoint.

Preheat the oven to 200°C/400°F/gas 6 and grease the baking tin.

In a food processor, pulse the lentils until they are blended. Add the almond butter, banana, cacao, honey and bicarbonate of soda and blend again, scraping down the sides to make sure everything is mixed together. Add the dates and blend again. Pour the mixture into the prepared tin and bake for 15 minutes. If it's gooey, that's good!

Let cool, slice into 12 bars and enjoy right away, dusted with cacao powder, or place in an airtight container in the fridge for up to 2 days.

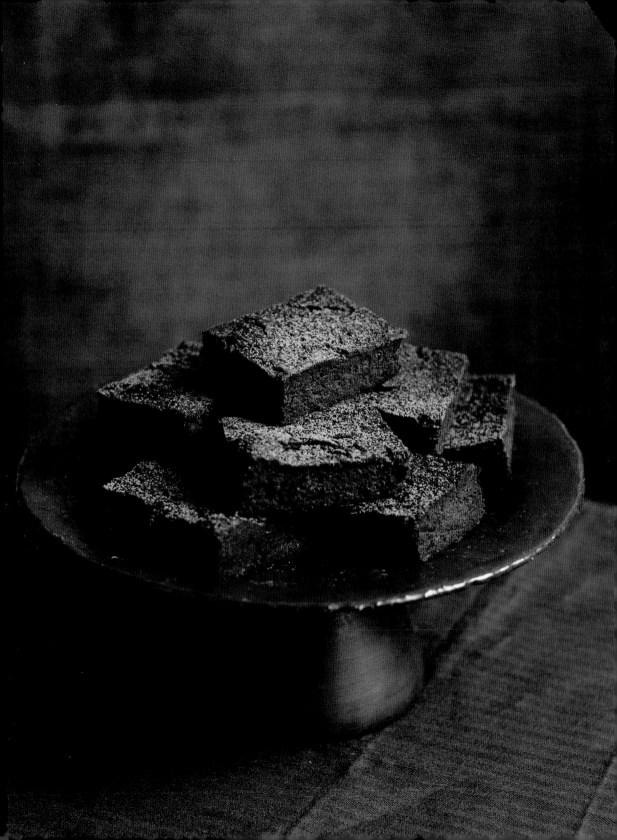

Honey Nut Blondies

2 tablespoons ground
  flaxseed (linseed), soaked in
  4 tablespoons warm water
50g (3 tablespoons + 1
  teaspoon) coconut oil, melted
100g (½ cup) coconut palm
  sugar
4 tablespoons honey
1 teaspoon sea salt
130g (1 cup) buckwheat flour
50g (heaping ⅓ cup) blanched
  almonds, roughly chopped
1 teaspoon vanilla extract

20 x 20-cm (8 x 8-inch)
  baking tin

Makes 12

My kids love these and I do to – maybe just a bit too
much, as I sometimes eat the whole batch! Most
shop-bought blondies are filled with a ton of refined
sugar and so here is a much healthier version that's
jam-packed with all things good!

Preheat the oven to 200°C/400°F/gas 6. Line the baking
tin with parchment paper.

In a medium bowl, add the flaxseed mixture, melted
coconut oil, coconut palm sugar, honey and salt and
mix well. Add the buckwheat flour and mix again.
Lastly, add the almonds and vanilla extract. Spread
the mixture evenly into the pan and bake for 15
minutes. The blondies will come out quite soft and
gooey but that, for me, makes them even better!

Cut into 12 bars and enjoy!

Cacao and Oat Dough Balls

No-Bake Chocolate Oat Bars

When my mum made chocolate chip cookies, I would plead with her to let me lick the bowl. Why? Because the dough was so, so good! But my mum also had a special way of baking the cookies. She took them out of the oven a couple of minutes early so that they'd be super soft, moist and practically like the dough from the bowl. Here's my version of semi-cooked dough balls – sweet, soft and super!

This recipe is a definite favourite of my kids', not only because the bars taste so good but also because they're super easy to make. I can actually give this recipe to any of my kids and they can whip it up in no time. It needs no baking! Incidentally, use any nuts you want. I've used walnuts and cashews, but almonds, pistachios and hazelnuts are all good choices, too!

120g (1 cup) oats
120g (1 cup) buckwheat flour
1 tablespoon melted coconut oil
6 Medjool dates, pitted and chopped
1 tablespoon honey
1 tablespoon maple syrup
1 tablespoon raw cacao powder
1 tablespoon ground flaxseed (linseed),
  soaked in 3 tablespoons warm water

100g (heaping ¾ cup) oats
75g (⅔ cup) cashews
65g (½ cup) walnut halves
1 tablespoon raw cacao powder
100ml (⅓ cup + 1 tablespoon) plant-based
  milk of your choice
3 tablespoons maple syrup
1 teaspoon vanilla extract

20 x 20-cm (8 x 8-inch) baking tin

Makes 24

Makes 12

Preheat the oven to 220°C/425°F/gas 7 and line a baking sheet with parchment paper.

In a bowl, mix together the oats and flour.

In another bowl, mix together the coconut oil, honey, maple syrup and cacao before adding in the flaxseed mixture. Stir well and then pour into the bowl with the oats and flour. Mix until everything combines together well and then tip in the dates.

Roll the mixture into 24 small balls and place on the prepared baking sheet. Bake for 10–12 minutes until the balls begin to brown and then remove them from the oven. Cool and serve.

Line the baking tin with parchment paper.

Put all the ingredients in a food processor and blend until well combined.

Spoon the mixture into the prepared baking tin and place in the freezer for 12 minutes to set. Remove and cut into 12 bars.

Matcha Chia Protein Squares

3 tablespoons chia seeds
60ml (¼ cup) coconut milk
  (or other plant-based milk
  of your choice)
135g (1 cup) oat flour (or just
  grind some rolled oats in a
  food processor)
3 tablespoons matcha powder,
  plus extra for dusting
1 teaspoon sea salt
120g (½ cup) almond butter
4 tablespoons honey
1 teaspoon vanilla extract

20 x 20-cm (8 x 8-inch)
  baking tin

Makes 16

These bars provide tons of energy and tons of protein, too! So at those times when you're having a slump in your day, or even in your week, whip these up and bring them with you wherever you go. The matcha will give you some major good-for-you energy and the chia seeds are packed with protein. Altogether a winning combination!

Soak the chia seeds in the coconut (or other plant-based) milk for 10 minutes. Meanwhile, line the baking tin with parchment paper.

In a large bowl, combine the oat flour, matcha and sea salt. Once mixed, add the almond butter, chia seed mixture, honey and vanilla. Stir well to combine (definitely use your hands!). Evenly press the mixture into the prepared tin and place in the freezer for 10 minutes to harden. Remove from the freezer and cut into 16 squares.

Eat straight away, dusted with a little matcha powder, or store in an airtight container in the fridge for up to a week.

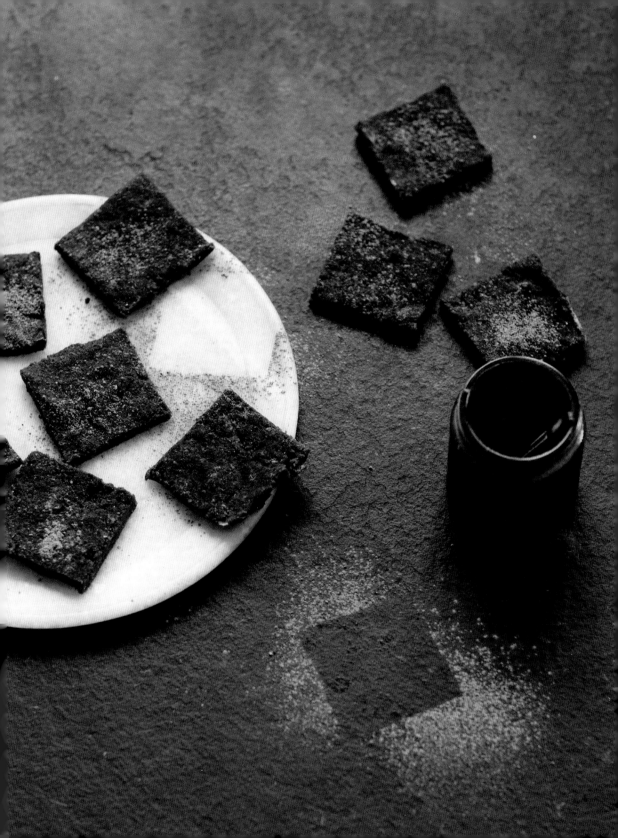

Crunchy Almond Butter Cookies

As you can probably tell from this cookbook, I love almond butter! Growing up in America, peanut butter cookies were all the rage. I don't even think I knew what almond butter was back then. But now, here we are, and almond butter is the new peanut butter! So, here's a healthy twist on a super classic.

150g (1½ cups) ground almonds
50g (scant ½ cup) buckwheat flour
4 tablespoons honey
4 tablespoons coconut oil, melted
3 tablespoons almond butter, plus a little extra for spreading, optional
1 tablespoon chia seeds, soaked in 3 tablespoons water
1 teaspoon ground cinnamon
¼ teaspoon baking powder

Makes about 12

Preheat the oven to 180°C/350°F/gas 4 and line a baking sheet with parchment paper.

Combine all the ingredients in a bowl, then use your hands to roll the mixture into 12 even-sized balls. Press each ball onto the prepared baking sheet, spacing them evenly apart. Bake for 10 minutes, then remove and allow to cool before eating.

These cookies are delicious with a little extra almond butter spread on top.

Goji Cinnamon Cookies

I love the smell of cookies baking in the oven and these ones don't hold back. You can literally smell the sweet scent of cinnamon while the cookies are rising. I like to think of these as not only delicious but a great way to incorporate more goji berries into your diet – and if you have kids, well, these go down a treat!

200g (1 cup) coconut palm sugar
1 large soft banana, mashed
2 tablespoons chia seeds, soaked in 6 tablespoons water for 5 minutes
4 tablespoons melted coconut oil
1 teaspoon vanilla extract
1 teaspoon lucuma powder
160g (1 cup) quinoa flour
½ teaspoon baking powder
½ teaspoon bicarbonate of soda (baking soda)
1 teaspoon ground cinnamon
30g (1oz) goji berries
120g (1 cup) oats

Makes 12–16

Preheat the oven to 200°C/400°F/gas 6 and line a baking sheet with parchment paper.

Combine the coconut palm sugar and banana in a large bowl. Mix in the chia seed gel, melted coconut milk, vanilla and lucuma powder. Stir in the flour, baking powder, bicarbonate of soda and ground cinnamon. Finally, add the goji berries and oats.

Using your hands, take small balls of the dough and press down into cookie shapes on the prepared baking sheet. Bake for 10 minutes or until golden brown.

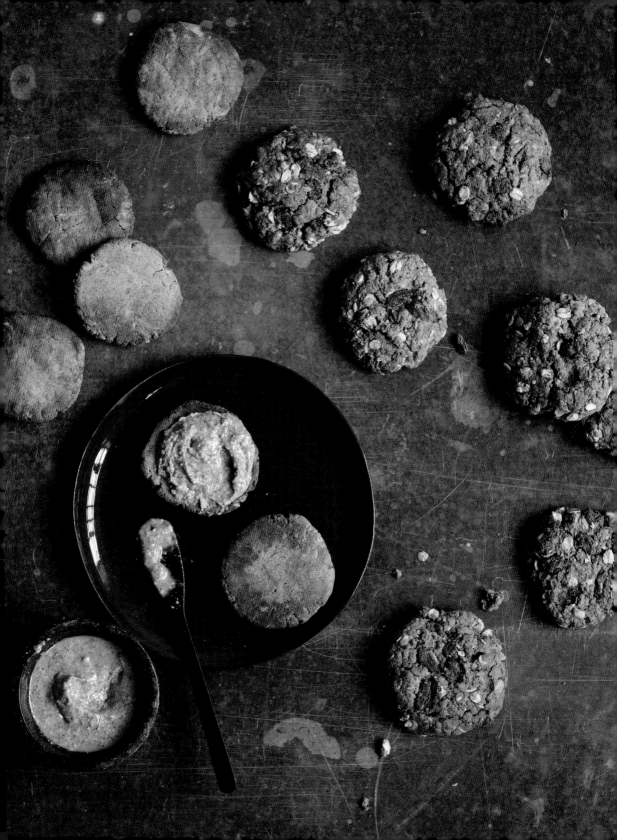

Banoffee Cups

2 large ripe bananas
16 Medjool dates, pitted
120g (1 cup) pecans, chopped
1 avocado, peeled and stoned
500ml (2 cups) coconut milk
4 tablespoons raw cacao
  powder
4 tablespoons cashew butter
4 ice cubes

Serves 4

End your meal on a high note with this dessert – it's so, so easy, but so, so good! And it's so, so healthy, too! If you need cheering up or you need to cheer someone else up, make this. There's no way a smile won't appear after just one spoonful!

Cut 4 slices of banana and 1 date into small slices and set aside with a few of the pecans. Blend all the rest of the ingredients in a food processor or blender until nicely smooth.

Spoon into cups or bowls and place in the freezer for 10 minutes to set. Top with the pecans and reserved banana slices and dates, and serve.

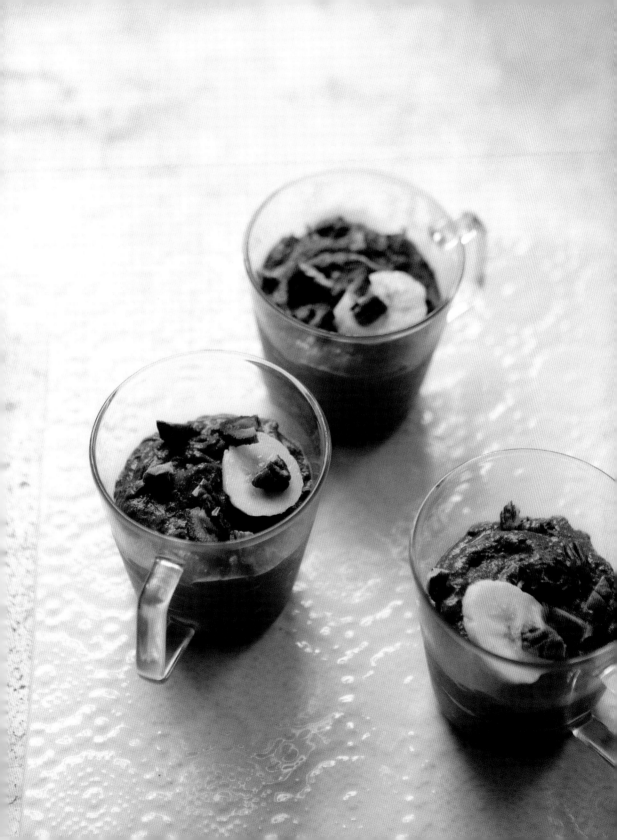

Sweets in Jars

I love serving meals in jars, as I just think it's really pretty and definitely different! But also, it's super easy to stack up the ingredients in the jars and wow your guests, especially if you need a quick dessert to serve. These recipes serve two, but it's very easy for you to multiply the ingredients to make more if needed. So, here are two delicious jar recipes from my supper guests to yours.

Chocolate Avocado Pudding Jar

1 banana
½ avocado, peeled and stoned
25g (¼ cup) ground almonds
4 tablespoons maple syrup
1 tablespoon raw cacao powder
1 teaspoon vanilla extract
1 teaspoon lucuma powder
½ tablespoon coconut oil

2 jam jars, cleaned and dried

Blitz all the ingredients into a creamy paste in a food processor or blender before spooning into the jars. Place in the freezer for 10 minutes to set before serving.

Sweet Fruit Salad Jar

4 tablespoons honey
1 banana, chopped
70g (½ cup) chopped pineapple
80g (½ cup) chopped mango
70g (½ cup) chopped strawberries
2 teaspoons chia seeds

2 jam jars, cleaned and dried

Spoon a tablespoon of honey into each jar, then divide the fruit equally between each and sprinkle with chia seeds. Finish off your jars with a last spoonful of honey and serve.

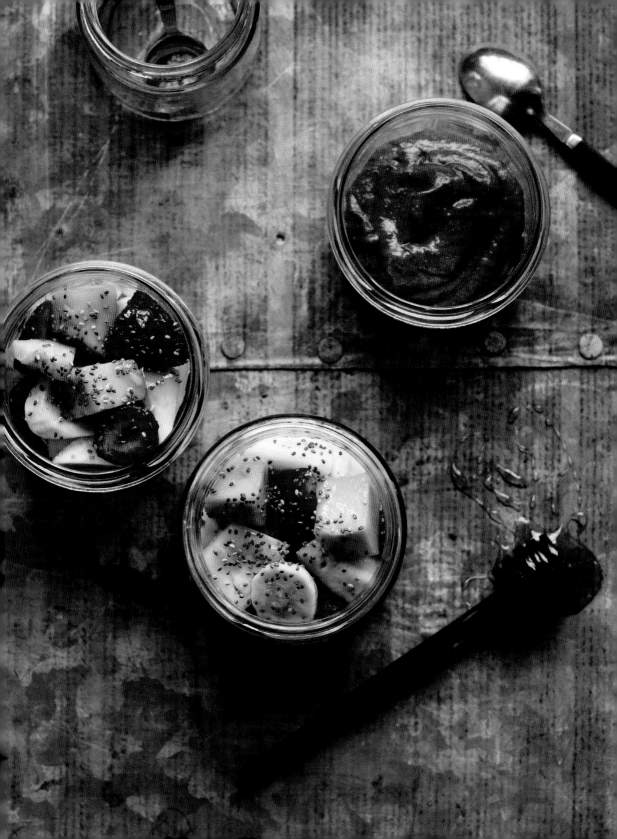

Peach and Rosemary Crumble

6 large ripe peaches, stoned and cut into small chunks or thinly sliced
90g (¾ cup) oats
60g (½ cup) buckwheat flour
5 rosemary sprigs, leaves separated
75ml (5 tablespoons) coconut oil, melted
55g (3 tablespoons + 2 teaspoons) coconut palm sugar
2 tablespoons honey or maple syrup
2 tablespoons arrowroot powder
1 teaspoon vanilla extract
½ teaspoon sea salt

baking dish, roughly 24 x 16cm (9½ x 6in)

Serves 6–8

I love this sweet dish, especially when peaches are in season. This is a truly delicious summer pudding, but any leftovers can be eaten for breakfast. No joke! Just add some almond milk and you have not only a super after-dinner sweet but a super sunrise, too!

Preheat the oven to 220°C/425°F/gas 7.

In a large bowl, mix all the ingredients together until well combined and crumbly. Spoon into the baking dish and bake for 15 minutes. The crumble will come out hot and bubbly and absolutely delicious!

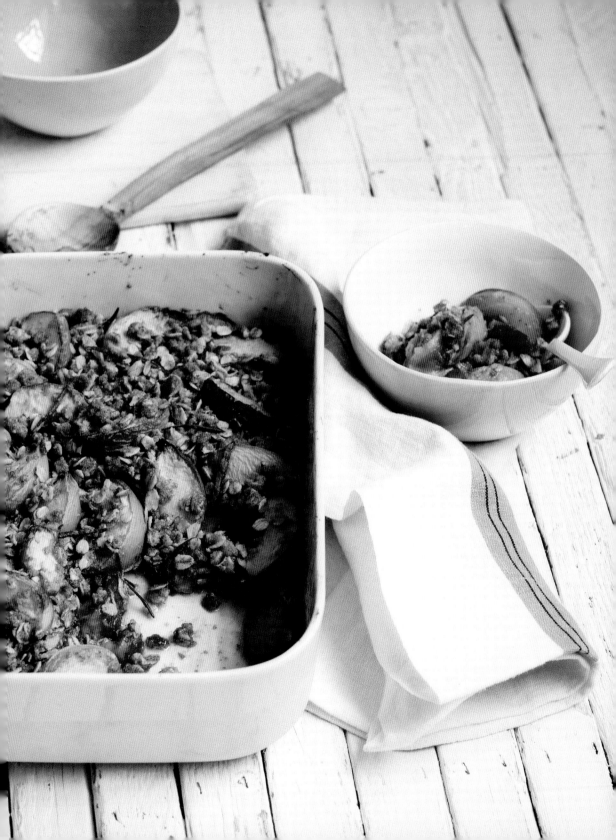

Creamy Chocolate Mylkshake

2 good-sized bananas
4 dates (Medjool are my
  favourite!), pitted
200ml (¾ cup) plant-based milk
100ml (½ cup) coconut milk
2 tablespoons raw cacao
  powder
1 tablespoon goji berries
1 teaspoon chia seeds
ice, optional

2 mini glass milk bottles or
  Kilner/Mason jars, cleaned
  and dried, and straws

Serves 2

My two youngest are obsessed with milkshakes and
I have to give credit where credit is due. This recipe
is all theirs. But it did take a lot of experimenting,
which meant a lot of mess to clear up! Thankfully they
found the perfect combination for the perfect Creamy
Chocolate Mylkshake.

Blitz all the ingredients in a food processor or blender
(with ice, if you prefer) and serve in mini retro milk
bottles or Kilner/Mason jars with straws.

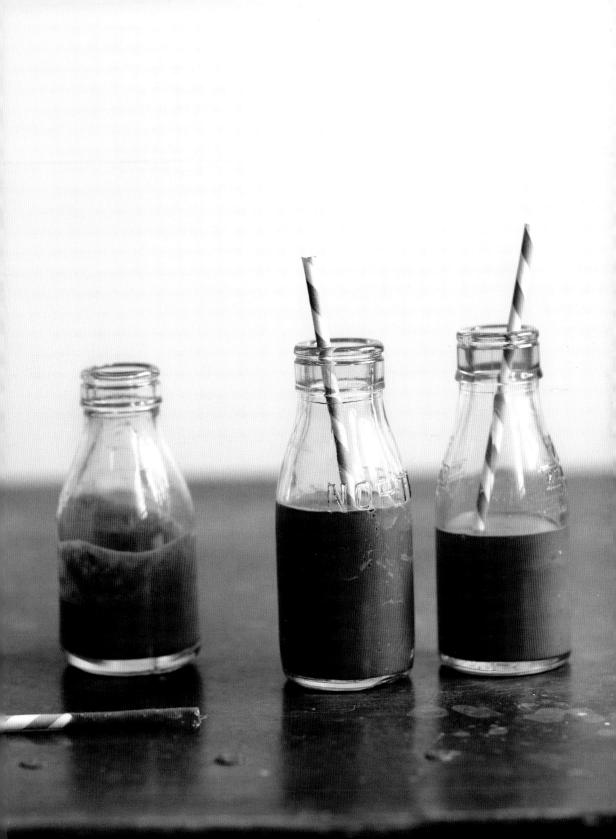

Index

For Emma, my SUPER girl

Acknowledgments

My journey to this point has been full of emotions, trials, failures (yes, plenty!) and some wonderful happy memories too. But as Arthur Ashe said: 'Success is a journey not a destination. The doing is usually more important than the outcome,' and this holds true to my path and this book. And for that, I want to say thank you to all of YOU who have followed me on my journey. I read every comment, email, post, and message on social media and in my inbox and I can't begin to tell you how grateful I am for all of your kind and inspiring words. Thank you. This book certainly wouldn't be here if it weren't for your love and support.

Thank you to my husband Luke and four kids, Emma, Jack, William and Nestor. We were shocked, surprised and thrilled when *Superfoods* came to fruition and even more elated when this book came around. 'Two cookbooks' is all I could say! All the hugs, screaming for joy, jumping around will be remembered forever.

Thank you to my wonderful sister-in-law Jemima for your constant support, loving words and simply being so caring. Oh, and your recipe in the book is very good, too!

Thank you, Alix Jones, for well, everything! I don't even know where to begin, but three years later and here we are. Thank you.

Thank you, Calgary Avansino, for being a huge inspiration in my journey to here and I look forward to our journeys colliding even more in the future.

Thank you, Rosemary Scoular and Aoife Rice, my wonderful agents, for believing in me and supporting me in all that I do. To Céline Hughes, my amazing editor, for making this follow-up to *Superfoods*, a Super Book Number 2! And thank you to the incredible team who helped put this book together again, Yuki, Iris, Nikki and Rebecca. From the yoga breaks during those long, dark winter days to the toasting with Japanese sake, I can't wait to do it again.

Thank you, Hannah Bryce, my publicist, for working over and beyond what any other publicist would do!

Finally, thank you to all of the incredible brands, and the people behind them, who have supported me, inspired me and rooted for me over the past several years. You know who you are. Thank you.

Publishing Director: Sarah Lavelle
Creative Director: Helen Lewis
Senior Editor: Céline Hughes
Senior Designer: Nicola Ellis
Photographer: Yuki Sugiura
Prop Stylist: Iris Bromet
Food Styling: Julie Montagu, Rebecca Woods
Production: Tom Moore, Vincent Smith

First published in 2016 by
Quadrille Publishing Limited
Pentagon House
52–54 Southwark Street
London SE1 1UN
www.quadrille.co.uk

Quadrille is an imprint of Hardie Grant
www.hardiegrant.com.au

Text © 2016 Julie Montagu
All photography © 2016 Yuki Sugiura
Design and layout © 2016 Quadrille
Publishing Limited

Cataloguing in Publication Data: a catalogue record for this book is available from the British Library.

ISBN: 978 184949 786 2

Printed in China